FOR THE PATIENT'S GOOD

FOR THE PATIENT'S GOOD

The Restoration of Beneficence in Health Care

EDMUND D. PELLEGRINO, M.D.

Director, Joseph and Rose Kennedy Institute for Ethics
John Carroll Professor of Medicine and Medical Humanities
Georgetown University Medical Center

DAVID C. THOMASMA, Ph.D.

Director, Medical Humanities Program
Fr. Michael I. English, S. J. Professor of Medical Ethics
Loyola University of Chicago Stritch School of Medicine

New York   Oxford
OXFORD UNIVERSITY PRESS
1988

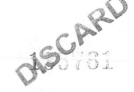

Oxford University Press

Oxford   New York   Toronto
Delhi   Bombay   Calcutta   Madras   Karachi
Petaling Jaya   Singapore   Hong Kong   Tokyo
Nairobi   Dar es Salaam   Cape Town
Melbourne   Auckland

and associated companies in
Beirut   Berlin   Ibadan   Nicosia

Published by Oxford University Press, Inc.,
200 Madison Avenue, New York, New York 10016

Oxford is a registered trademark of Oxford University Press

Library of Congress Cataloging-in-Publication Data
Pellegrino, Edmund D., 1920–
For the patient's good.
Bibliography: p.
Includes index.
1. Medical ethics.   2. Benevolence.   3. Physician and patient.
I. Thomasma, David C., 1939–   .   II. Title.
[DNLM: 1. Ethics, Medical. 2. Physician-Patient Relations. W 62 P386f]
R725.5.P45   1988   174′.2   87-15214
ISBN 0-19-504319-7

3 5 7 9 8 6 4 2

Printed in the United States of America
on acid-free paper

*To our parents, wives, and families
—who have nurtured our work through their
patience and devotion*

Preface

Every participant in clinical ethical decisions—physician, patient, family, surrogate, guardian, the court—invokes the good of the patient to justify his or her moral choice. But as soon as we ask what we mean by the patient's good, who is to determine it, and by what criteria and procedures, we run into controversy, both in theory and in practice.

Is the patient's good equated simply with his or her medical needs, with his or her own interpretation of what is good, or with what the doctor judges to be good medicine? Who determines what is good when the definitions of the participants in the decision are in conflict? How does the good of the patient relate to social and economic good? What do we mean by the good doctor? By the good patient? By good medicine?

This book examines the notion of the patient's good from a philosophical and practical point of view. It seeks a more explicit understanding of the ancient principle of beneficence and its actual and supposed conflict with the principles of autonomy and justice. It proposes to locate the proper place of beneficence in the reconstruction of the ethics of the profession of medicine that is currently in progress.

We will contend that beneficence remains the central moral principle in the ethics of medicine, that it entails more than the negative principle *primum non nocere,* and that it entails positive enhancement of all the components packed into the complex notion of the patient's good.

We argue that the patient seeks not only to be protected from harm, but also to be healed and to have health restored or improved, pain and anxiety relieved, disability lessened. The patient desires these good ends within some definition of the good life that is uniquely and personally his or her own. In this view medical or technical good is assuredly one indispensable component. But true healing goes beyond strictly medical values to embrace the moral and other values of the patient.

Our aim is to redefine, and refine, the notion of beneficence in terms of the new practicalities and dimensions of the physician-patient relationship today. With the recent emergence in medical ethics of the principle of autonomy, it seems necessary to strike a new balance between autonomy and beneficence, which to some ethicists seem to be in conflict.

This is an especially crucial relationship in our morally polyglot society. Physicians, families, and patients often arrive at radically different interpretations of what is in the best interests of a particular patient, at a particular time, and in a particular clinical situation. An essential step in defining these differences, comprehending their origins, and dealing with them in morally sustainable ways is to unpack the notion of patient good. This is the proximate end of all clinical-ethical decisions, and it shapes the other decisions that lead up to it.

In an earlier work, *A Philosophical Basis of Medical Practice,* we proposed that the special nature of the doctor-patient relationship should be the source of the canons of professional medical ethics, complementing or even replacing a rights ethic.[1] We based our contention on the notion that health is a good and an end in medicine. In the present work we develop that notion further, showing how it undergirds an ethic of loyalty to the patient, social obligations, compassion, and the characteristics or virtues that should govern the healing relationship. A rights ethic, to our thinking, is a minimalist ethic. An ethic based on beneficence embraces more fully the nuances of the patient's best interests.

Even though specific ethical and biomedical ethical issues are discussed in all our chapters, our primary concern is to continue the search for a coherent philosophy of medicine. This book is written for colleagues interested in the ways in which philosophy, ethics, and medicine relate to each other, and for those who find deficiencies in contemporary medical moral theories. It is also written for all health professionals, practicing physicians, nurses, and allied health professionals, as well as lawyers and policymakers. We hope they will find insights that apply to their professions as well as to medicine. Since we have the temerity to speak of the "good of the patient" and even the "good patient," we also hope the general public will read this book, for we almost all become patients eventually.

Despite some changes in our views since the publication of our first book, one theme remains unchanged—that is, that, along with the currently dominant ethical theories based on individual rights and duties or social utilities, there stands a third theory. This is an ethics based on a theory of the good, in this instance the patient's good. This theory appeared in our earlier work, in which we argued that medicine is neither a science nor an art, but a practice that gives rise to ethical axioms. If these axioms are violated, the good of medicine would also be violated.

This book is divided into three sections. In the first we develop a model of the doctor-patient relation as "beneficence-in-trust." In the second we examine the implications of this model for that relationship. In the third we present in detail some consequences of the beneficence model with respect to the difficult challenges facing health care (allocation of resources, the physician as gate-keeper, decisions about incompetent patients, and so on), paying special attention to the ways in which our proposal leads us to different conclusions than others, even some courts, have drawn.

We close with an attempt to summarize the moral obligations that derive from the concept of patient good in an explicit declaration of obligations. We offer this statement of commitments as a step toward reconstituting existing professional codes we deem necessary in contemporary society. We believe this statement of commitments is applicable to all health professionals, not simply physicians.

We are cognizant of our boldness in thus amplifying and modifying the ancient and recent codes of professional ethics. We make our proposal humbly and hopefully—not as a final or apodictic codification, but as a stimulus to further thought and discussion.

We are deeply grateful to our secretaries, Marti Patchell and Kay Cahill Scarano, for their tireless devotion in typing and retyping the many drafts of this manuscript. Jo Ann Immekus, David G. Miller, Ginny Fallon, Eric Janney, and John Guardi also deserve our thanks for their assistance in this task. Our research assistants, Virginia Ashby Sharpe and John P. McNulty, spent many hours with the manuscript in its successive versions. Their dedication exceeds our ability properly to thank them.

Washington, D.C.　　　　　　　　　　　　　　　　　　　E.D.P.
Chicago, Illinois　　　　　　　　　　　　　　　　　　　D.C.T.
April 1987

Contents

I

THE DELINEATION OF BENEFICENCE

1

Paternalism, Autonomy, and Beneficence in the Doctor-Patient Relationship

Two major ethical theories are today vying for dominance in medical ethics. The first, inherited from the Enlightenment, stresses the liberty and autonomy of the individual. It gathered strength in the nineteenth century in response to the depreciation of personal worth that accompanied the Industrial Revolution. This theory grounds ethics in rights, duties, and obligations. The second theory stresses social utility rather than individual autonomy. Ironically, it too gained ascendancy during the Industrial Revolution to counter the social atomism of a purely individualistic ethic. This theory stresses social good, rules of conduct, and social accountability. Mill laid the foundation for such theories when he proposed the principle of autonomy, on the one hand, and the principle of utility, on the other.

Applied to the physician-patient relationship, the first theory imposes on the physician the obligation of respect for the patient's self-determination.[1] The second theory requires that the physician act to maximize benefits and goods even if this might demand acting without the patient's consent. It sanctions overriding the patient's autonomous decision if that decision is not judged by the physician to be in the patient's or society's good.

We intend to show in this chapter that an older, third theory based on beneficence, that is, on acting for the good of the patient, and on virtue is more appropriate to the special context of the medical encounter today. This theory was originally formulated by Socrates, Plato, and Aristotle, reinforced by the Roman Stoics, and modified by Saint Thomas Aquinas. It is the theory that prevailed in Western culture until Enlightenment, when it came under attack by the French philosophers and the British empiricists.[2]

The reintroduction of an ethics based on beneficence and virtue requires modification and reinterpretation in much the same way that Dewey developed his theory of character as a solution to the clash between deontology and utilitarianism.[3] We address this task in the following way in this chapter: first, by tracing the background of recent dissatisfaction with medical paternalism and autonomy; second, by examining the need for a reassessment of models of the physician-patient relationship; and, third, by discussing a definition of the terms used in the book. This serves as a prolegomenon to our discussion of the limitations of autonomy and paternalism in the next chapter.

BACKGROUND

Almost weekly some columnist expounds at length, and with passion, on the insensitivity to the patient's wishes he or she perceives in the way physicians treat their patients. For example, Gloria Chaines, a free-lance writer for the Chicago *Tribune,* had this to say: "They have us cornered in the medical marketplace, their arrogance unwarranted, their lack of sensitivity insufferable, and I don't like it one bit." She goes on to chide physicians because "asking for a plausible explanation is still scorned as presumptuous. Many doctors talk to patients as though they were slightly retarded, deliberately creating a condition of dependency."[4]

Allowing for a certain amount of journalistic license, Chaines' opinion accurately expresses the perceptions of many ethicists, lawyers, and the public about the way physicians ignore their patients' rights and their desires for understanding, and participation in, the decisions that affect them.

The legal right to refuse treatment is firmly grounded in the right to privacy, or, as Justice Brandeis termed it, the right to be left alone. The President's Commission for the Study of Ethical Problems in Medicine and Biomedical and Behavioral Research reasserted that right: "Adults are entitled to accept or reject health care interventions on the basis of their personal values and in furtherance of their personal goals."[5]

The overwhelming acceptance of this legal right of privacy has coincided with social and political trends to make participatory democracy, distrust of authority, and acceptance of moral pluralism in other spheres characteristic of American life. The result, especially in the last two decades, has been to undermine the twenty-five-hundred-year-old Hippocratic model of the physician as the benign, authoritarian, paternalistic decision maker, taking the full responsibility for the welfare of his or her patient. According to the Hippocratic oath, the physician promises to "follow that system of regimen which according to my ability and judgment I consider for the benefit of my patients." Nowhere in the Hippocratic corpus is there any provision for the patient's view of things. In fact, in one place the relationship is described as being between "one who orders and one who obeys."[6]

Undoubtedly, there have always been isolated instances of patient dissent from this authoritarian view of the physician's role. Also, in U.S. law the principle of privacy has for some time been asserted in support of the patient's legal right to refuse treatment even in life-threatening situations. But the most influential test of this traditional, paternalistic model of the patient-doctor relationship occurred in the *Karen Ann Quinlan* case.[7] In that case the Supreme Court of New Jersey ruled that the state's interests (and medical interests) in keeping a person alive are superseded in irreversible situations by a person's wishes—in this case Quinlan's previously expressed wish not to remain on a life-support system such as a respirator.

What is often forgotten is that the hospital and physicians in charge of Quinlan's care did not accept this judgment. They still considered removal of the respirator to be "murder," since Quinlan's brain waves were not flat. In effect, the physicians did not accept the argument or the court's authority that the patient (or proxy) is the ultimate arbiter of the patient's own good.

Their refusal, at first blush, seems at odds with a patient's rights perspective, confirming the worst kind of paternalism. It certainly appears, in retrospect, to violate the explicit letter, if not the spirit, of more recent legislation designed to make it clear that the authority to treat comes from the patient. Consider, for example, the wording of the House Enrolled Act No. 1830, Section F, of the Indiana General Assembly:

> All patients or clients are entitled to be informed of the nature of treatment or habilitation program proposed, the known effects of receiving and of not receiving such treatment or habilitation, and alternative treatment or habilitation programs, if any. An adult voluntary patient or client, if not adjudicated incompetent, is entitled to refuse to submit to treatment or to a habilitation program and is entitled to be informed of this right.[8]

To many, including physicians, it is a puzzle why Quinlan's doctors could not accept the judgment of the New Jersey Supreme Court. So strongly has the emphasis on rights and autonomy in medical ethics prevailed that Quinlan's doctors, adhering to their interpretation of an earlier notion of beneficence, found themselves acting contrary to public and professional opinion. This is a situation that would not have occurred a few decades ago.

The sources for this sort of resistance to medical paternalism are many: the political and ethical philosophy of individual rights;[9] the higher educational level of today's public; the latter's awareness of the powers and dangers of medical technology; a distrust of experts; the rise of consumerism; and the moral challenges of the Vietnam War, the civil rights movement, and the campus revolts of the sixties and early seventies. The convergence of these forces has been powerful enough to erode the twenty-five-hundred-year-old tradition of medical status contained in beneficent authoritarianism.

The challenge these forces have brought against traditional medical paternalism are, in our view, often well founded. The resulting enhancement of the patient's participation in clinical decisions is to our minds a salubrious development.[10] What concerns us—and what is significant for medical ethics in both its individual and its societal manifestations—is a growing potentiality for conflict between the moral obligation to autonomy and the moral obligation to beneficence, and the almost automatic assumption of some ethicists and patients that autonomy must always supervene.[11]

To accord autonomy superiority over beneficence is sometimes to abandon the patient in time of need.[12] It is readily admitted by advocates of the autonomy model that in the case of a comatose or otherwise incompetent patient, acting on his or her behalf is not a form of paternalism,[13] or of "weak" paternalism at best. In terms of legal rights as well, the right to self-determination may be overridden on grounds of beneficence when one's competence is impaired for some reason.[14] If the physician made no effort to assess the patient's competency, or to dissuade a competent but noncompliant or obtuse patient from an ill-conceived decision, then the patient's autonomy would block the care the physician should have for his patient. It could result in actual harm to the patient.

In any given interpretation of the concern we should show for other persons in general or in a medical context, the question of the degree to which interference would be permissible remains a difficult one to answer. To determine not to intervene is a form of passive cooperation with possibly harmful actions. Such cooperation cannot be excused with a simple assertion of the principle of autonomy. The physician-patient covenant—if we accept such a model of the relationship—does not provide for the notion of freely contracting individuals. The covenantal model is phenomenologically opposed to the Lockean model of a contract. In a Lockean model two or more autonomous entities form a bond for some mutual good. In a covenantal model the bond is formed based on the need of one party.

We agree with Cassell that a task of medicine is to restore autonomy, and with Newton that the concern for autonomy must be tempered by the realities of the impact of disease on patients.[15] Nevertheless, there are weaknesses in both the autonomy and paternalism models when they are applied to a relationship as complex as the medical relationship. Paternalism overrides the dignity and humanity of the patient; autonomy overrides the concern we should show for helping each other, especially if we belong to a group ordained by society specifically to help in the special human circumstances we call illness.

REASSESSMENT OF THE PHYSICIAN-PATIENT RELATIONSHIP

We argued in our first book that the philosophical foundation of medical ethics is grounded in the nature of the patient-physician relationship. For those who abhor the use of the term *nature,* we would substitute the term *model.* The richness, variety, and complexity of the healing relationship are reflected in the differences we perceive in the many models that purport to define how doctors and patients relate in the medical enterprise.

Some propose a "biological" model, others a contractual, economic, or religious model.[16-18] The first three models reduce the complexity of the human relationship to some conveniently simpler mode—each of which is a factor in the relationship but none of which is sufficient to define the whole of that relationship. The Hippocratic model, on the other hand, errs on the side of pretentiousness. We acknowledge the real importance of the religious dimensions of medical care but remain convinced that this is not synonymous with a hieratic role for the physician.[19]

Except for the hieratic model, the newer models have been elaborated more to counter the excesses of the traditional paternalistic model than to reexamine the whole relationship with a view to reconstructing a medical ethic that is sensitive to both autonomy and beneficence without absolutizing either paternalism or autonomy. We can, we believe, admit that the paternalistic model is antiquated without repudiating everything bequeathed to us by the long tradition of physician beneficence.[20]

Our own proposal is grounded in a conviction that a professional ethic based on the existential situation of the patient is apt to be a more reliable guide than one based simply on the assertion and counterassertion of ethical principles.[21] We will enlarge on the model in subsequent chapters. Before we do make such a proposal, however, we must define some key terms and then provide a critique of the shortcomings of both the autonomy and the beneficence models as they are currently construed. This will involve defining the key terms *paternalism, autonomy,* and—parenthetically, because of the orientation of our own proposal—*healing.* The critique will occur in the next chapter.

Paternalism

Paternalism centers on the notion that the physician—either by virtue of his or her superior knowledge or by some impediment incidental to the patient's experience of illness—has better insight into the best interests of the patient than does the patient, or that the physician's obligations are such that he is impelled to do what is medically good, even if it is not "good" in terms of the patient's own value system.[22,23]

Paternalism occurs in two forms, strong and weak. Strong paternalism consists in overriding the competent wishes and choices of another. For example, the doctor in the movie *Whose Life Is It Anyway?* gives his patient a sedative against the latter's expressed wish.[24] Today this form of paternalism is far less prevalent than previously, though it still persists in certain situations and among certain physicians.

Far more common is weak paternalism, an action taken in the best interests of a patient who cannot give a fully informed consent for some reason, or who is not afforded the full possibility of free choice. Thus, the physician may decide in advance what treatment he considers is in the patient's best interests. He then presents only this option, or so shapes the information he provides that this is the only choice the patient could make.

Ackerman has argued that weak paternalism of this kind is justifiable in some instances of research involving children.[25] Dworkin argues that some limited forms of paternalism might be regarded as a king of "social insurance policy" that rational persons might take out to protect themselves under previously agreed upon conditions.[26] An example might be the presumption to treat every patient brought to the emergency room. Here the anxiety, urgency, uncertainty, the emotional stresses might be such that fully competent decisions could be precluded for a significant number of patients and their families.

Since, according to Dworkin's formulation, there would be prior agreement on the presumption to treat, this would not be paternalism at all but a form of negotiated beneficence. Likewise, if the patient cannot give consent because of coma, mental retardation, or shock, or if the physician cannot ascertain the patient's wishes from others, he may presume to act on his own interpretation of the patient's interests. Under these circumstances paternalism loses its derogatory implications and is subsumed under beneficence. Childress makes some affirmative distinctions such as direct and indirect, active and passive. These are important but not directly relevant to our argument.

Autonomy

The term *autonomy* stems from the Greek for "self-rule" or "self-law." Kant made the concept the dowel pin of his moral theory by proposing that the self, through duty, is the legitimate origin of law. Similarly, John Stuart Mill proposed that a person cannot interfere with the freedom of others unless they cause harm to others or act out of ignorance.[27]

In his highly regarded exploration of the concept, Dworkin argued that autonomy entailed authenticity and independence, that is, freedom of action (independence) and motives for action that were one's own (authenticity).[28] Cassell used this concept effectively to argue that the proper object of medicine is to reestablish the patient's autonomy.[29]

Paternalism as Problematic

From the point of view of our thesis, the concept of autonomy is less problematic than the concept of paternalism. It is essential to examine some of the narrower definitions of paternalism put forward by today's ethicists. Their definitions predetermine, to some extent, their stance on the moral permissiveness of paternalism. Thus, Culver and Gert detect conflicting meanings in Childress' definition.[30] Buchanan's definition is considered too narrow regarding the kinds of moral rules that are violated.[31] Dworkin's is too dependent on legal cases and narrower still in its inclusion of coercion and interference with liberty.

Childress himself disagrees with Dworkin's narrow definition of paternalism as "roughly the interference with a person's liberty of action justified by reasons referring exclusively to the welfare, good, happiness, needs, interests or values of the person being coerced."[32] As Childress argues, "The issues of paternalism, particularly in health care, are broader than coercion, especially legal coercion."[33] Nonetheless, as we shall see, Childress does adopt a notion of "interference" with wishes as central to the idea of paternalistic acts.

One's definitions predetermine one's analyses. For example, we note that Childress' own definition of paternalism leads him to disagree with Gert and Culver, who hold that paternalism necessarily includes a violation of a moral rule (and thus always requires justification). Childress holds that paternalism is composed of "altruistic beneficence" toward persons, coupled with a refusal to respect their wishes.[34] He therefore argues that:

> it is both unnecessary and misleading to insist that the violation of moral rules is a condition of paternalism. It is unnecessary because it is sufficient to point to the refusal to acquiesce in a person's wishes, choices, or actions. It is misleading because it does not identify in specific terms what is common to all paternalistic acts, namely, this refusal to acquiesce in a person's wishes, choice, and actions.[35]

The problem with this argument about terms is that Culver and Gert do not share Childress' views on the relative importance of autonomy or respect for persons. They disagree with his emphasis on the weights that must be given to rights over duties. Hence they do not agree that the essence of paternalism is not respecting the wishes of another for that person's own good. Rather, they hold that the essence of paternalism lies in *unjustifiably* overriding the wishes of another—precisely the point at issue between them.

One may assume that Culver and Gert do not hold that every wish of the patient is to be honored, or even is honorable as such. Apparently, for Childress it must be thus, leading to his ranking of beneficence below autonomy in his writings, at least until 1985 (as we shall see in Chapter 4). Further, one wonders why this ranking does take place, given the fact that Childress so clearly distinguishes between the beneficent component of paternalism and the interference component. If one does not interfere with the patient's wishes, then "altruistic beneficence" should rise above all other considerations as a central feature of medicine.

Indeed, Childress does recognize that beneficence involves roles and relationships, particularly those in the doctor-patient relationship.[36] Yet this recognition leads to an entirely different concern from that of our own work. Childress notes that "both the language of physicians' duties [in such relationships], in contrast to patients' rights, and the content of those duties tend to be paternalistic, for they appear to allow and even to require the professional to determine the relevance and weights of benefits and harms to the patient."[37] But why must this be so? According to Childress' own thinking, beneficent altruism, without interference, does not necessarily lead to paternalistic duties. Once again, there is a subtle misidentification of paternalism with beneficence. In other words, Childress still thinks less of "beneficent altruism" in medicine than he does of "autonomy."

Because we do value beneficence in medicine at least as much as autonomy, we agree with Culver and Gert that what counts in paternalism is the unjustifiable overturning of patient wishes. Yet we find, in the case of Childress, that one cannot truly heal, that is, help a person become whole again, if one neglects, ignores, countermands, or destroys patient autonomy. Our focus, then, is on consent.

For the purposes of this book, paternalism should be understood to mean a medical decision to benefit a patient without full consent of the latter. Although fully informed consent is a theoretical ideal, the amount of information patients receive should be reasonably complete so that they can make a truly informed choice about treatment. Most paternalistic acts violate the reasonable information criterion on two counts. First, an action may need justification if the patient is competent to give consent, because the action might violate a moral rule, such as truth-telling (strong paternalism). Or, second, an action may need some justification if the patient is not fully competent to give consent due to age or mental status (weak paternalism).

Healing

We have defined the end goal of medicine as a right and good healing action for a particular patient.[38] Throughout this work we will use the term *healing* in a way that requires some operational definition.

We have already mentioned that healing involves more than a cure. The aim of medicine is to address not only the bodily assault that disease or an injury inflicts but also the psychological, social, even spiritual dimensions of this assault. To heal is to make whole or sound, to help a person reconvene the powers of the self and return, as far as possible, to his conception of a normal life. Many physicians today stress the integrity of the body, soul, and spirit in healing.[39] The process of healing involves at least four levels or stages: pain; provisional recovery of wholeness; sloughing off dead tissue or past constructions; and regeneration.[40] These stages occur at biological, personal, and social levels.

By stressing healing, we do not wish to downgrade the effort to cure a disease, for most often a truly effective treatment is supposed to assist the sick person back to normalcy. But when curing is not possible—as when a patient suffers a terminal disease, or when a degenerative disease such as Alzheimer's is present, the therapeutic activity of medicine need not cease.

The primary meaning of healing, however, is to make the body sound. In our previous work we defined medicine as an art of healing that primarily works in and through the body to achieve integration of the lived world of the patient. Even if one is incurably ill, dying, in pain or distress, it is possible, in some measure at least, to restore a sense of balance, an integration of meaning and living.[41]

Protecting autonomy is an important ethical principle because it provides a key way to respect persons. Traditionally, its contrasting principle, paternalism, was also seen as a way to respect the value of persons. We turn next to an exploration of weaknesses of the patient autonomy and medical paternalism models for the practice of medicine.

2

Limitations of Autonomy and Paternalism: Towards a Model of Beneficence

Three radical changes have occurred in the ancient edifice of medical ethics in the last two decades. Each promises to transform the nature of the physician-patient relationship and lead to repercussions in the domains of law, society, and ethics. Each merits the most careful scrutiny by the profession and the public, because how we resolve the moral dilemmas they produce will determine not only public relationships with the medical profession, but what kind of society we are, or wish to be.

The three changes we consider most crucial are these: (1) the shift in the locus of decision making from the physician to the patient—a philosophical shift from the primacy of beneficence to the primacy of autonomy in physician-patient relationships; (2) an unprecedented expansion of medical technological capability, thus expanding enormously the range and complexity of clinical and policy decision in health care; and (3) the entry of economic considerations as primary forces in individual and policy decisions regarding health and medical care, thereby creating a conflict between the canon of economics and the canon of traditional medical ethics.

In this chapter we will confine ourselves to the first of this triad of changes—the shift from beneficence to autonomy in medical ethics. We recognize the interdependence of the whole traid of changes and acknowledge that dissecting them from each other is difficult and somewhat misleading. Yet the scope of this chapter prohibits a full examination of the interdependence of autonomy, technological possibility, and economics in the evolution of contemporary medical ethics.

This chapter consists of three parts: Initially, we will examine the limitations of the autonomy model of the physician-patient relationship. Next, we will examine the limitations of the paternalistic model. Finally, we will outline a model of beneficence that promotes the good of the patient while deabsolutizing autonomy and avoiding the pitfalls of traditional paternalism.

THE AUTONOMY MODEL AND ITS LIMITATIONS

Sociohistorical Critique of Autonomy

The autonomy model of clinical decision making is firmly grounded in the dignity of human persons and the claim they have on each other to privacy, self-direction, the establishment of their own values and life plans based on information and reasoning, and the freedom to act on the results of their cogitations. The historical origin of the principle of autonomy, as it is interpreted by many ethicists today, is of recent date. It is found mainly in the philosophical treatises of the French and English Enlightenment and the emergence of the doctrines of individual and political rights to freedom that undergird modern democracy.

The notions of individual rights and autonomy have been gathering strength in American public life since the founding of our country. They lagged behind in the medical relationship, however. Only in the last several decades have they become powerful enough to challenge the traditional paternalism that dominated the relations of doctors and patients for twenty-five-hundred years—at least since the time of Hippocrates.[1] For our purposes we need not trace this history in detail. It suffices to take note of the major forces that have nurtured the exponential growth of autonomy in the last two decades.

First is the expansion of political democracy to every sphere of civic life, fostering in each of us the desire to participate in the decisions that affect our lives as individuals. This "democratization" carries with it a certain distrust of all authority, expertise, privilege, and prerogative of the kind traditionally wielded by physicians, lawyers, and other professionals.

To this we must add the general improvement in the education of the public and the dissemination by the media of information about both the advances of medicine and the ethical and legal dilemmas those advances produce. As a result, the public appreciates that the decisions doctors make in the use of medical knowledge make a vast difference in our lives, and that those decisions increasingly involve value choices.

Lastly, the increasingly divergent moral pluralism in our society impels us to seek to protect our personal values against usurpation by others. This is recognized as a genuine danger in medical decisions, which can involve our deepest convictions about life and death, abortion, euthanasia, genetic manipulation, and the like.

These factors have converged to undermine the traditional model of the benign, paternalistic physician who assumes full responsibility and authority to

determine the patient's best interests and to act so as to advance those interests—if need be, without the patient's participation.[2] This is the conception of
beneficence still dominant in the minds of many physicians and patients; it still
shapes the ethos and ethics of medicine. It is the conception, too, that is the
focus of criticism by proponents of autonomy who equate beneficence almost
entirely with medical paternalism.

It is true that, here and there in the history of medicine, there were suggestions of patient participation in clinical decisions. Plato, for example, distinguished the physician of the free man from the physician of the slave by the fact
that the former educated and consulted with his patient, while the latter did not.
It is true, too, as Katz points out, that in more recent times, some such as de
Dorbière tentatively suggest that patients ought to be part of the doctor's decisions.[3] Moreover, a closer reading of Percival's *Ethics* serves to qualify the standard account of the eighteenth-century physician as merely a condescending
gentleman-authoritarian.[4] The same is true of some aspects of Hooker's work on
physicians and patients, an American work on medical morals that deserves to
be better known.[5]

But exceptions like these aside, paternalism was the dominant, and indeed
the accepted, model of the clinical relationship for most of medicine's history.
Paternalism was not as ethically dubious in times past as it is today. For one
thing, the educational gap between physician and patient was wider than it is
now. Further, participatory democracy, even in Greek times, was not a reality
for most people. Finally, almost all medical treatments were nonspecific, as
much dependent upon faith in the physician as on any genuine therapeutic
potency. Indeed, most therapeutic efforts were either useless or dangerous. Ordinary patients were not aware, however, of the therapeutic poverty of most
prescriptions.

"Aesculapian power" was a major ingredient of cure. It rested on faith in
the quasi-hieratic power and authority of the physician as a person. Indeed, the
physician was part and parcel of the cure, as Lain-Entralgo points out.[6,7] Only in
recent times have these conditions changed so radically that the more objectionable features of medical paternalism have begun to be felt. Medicine's capacities
to alter individual and social life are unprecedented. An educated public grasps
this fact, and no image grants the physician unrestricted discretion in the use of
his powers.

Freidson has detailed the negative effects of the professionalization of contemporary medicine.[8] His study is very cogent, but it undervalues some of the
more positive aspects of professionalization. Anything so powerful as modern
medicine requires a formal professionalization process to assure that high levels
of competence, conduct, and accountability are maintained. This aspect of professionalization must not be lost in the current antipathy to paternalism.

In fact, the dangers of paternalism lie less in professionalization than in irre-
sponsible uses of power and the attributions of superiority that arise from the
social ascendancy of medicine. As Mill remarked, "Whenever there is an ascendant class, a large portion of the morality emanates from its class interests and

its feelings of superiority."[9] This is the basis for Illich's mordant criticism, too, but he weakens his case by the polemics of social revolution with which he heavily flavors his charges against medicine.[10]

Thus, the revulsion many competent adults feel about medical paternalism may more properly derive from anger about physicians' pretensions as a superior class than from any inherent property of professionalism itself. Feminists have argued that sexism and patriarchial values show up in gyneocologists' trivialization of womens' complaints—for example, the premenstrual syndrome debate. Patients are forced to wait for the doctor in the antechamber, suggesting that their time, their values, and their lives are not as important as the doctor's. Cartoons abound in which the public fears that doctors are too busy managing their money to care about patients. These are examples more of the role of power and class than of any inherent properties of professionalization. They are often at the root of the declining status of the physician as recorded in serial American Medical Association (AMA) surveys on the public image of the profession.[11]

The patient autonomy movement is an understandable counterreaction to such class domination. Nonetheless, autonomy should not be viewed as an absolute model for the doctor-patient relationship itself because it is insufficient to claim, as the move to patient autonomy often does, that medical paternalism is a direct outgrowth of professionalization. Nor is paternalism a prima facie medical or social evil, as Berlant supposes.[12] Modern medicine incorporates moments of patient choice as well as moments of necessary, beneficial paternalism. The former occur when the diagnosis and options are clear and well documented. The latter occur when not enough is known about a disease and its prognosis, when no therapeutic modality has a clear edge, or when an existing therapy has marginal or dubious benefit. In these cases physicians may be forced to recommend, or even urge, a course of action based on an intuitive assessment of the data. The important thing here is that the physician make clear the uncertainties with which he or she must contend. This preserves autonomy and so is not paternalistic but beneficent.

Some philosophers who defend the absoluteness of patient autonomy on moral grounds neglect the fact that "decision making" among humans is an interpersonal transaction. They thus downgrade the bilaterality of the physician-patient relationship. Doctor and patient are existentially bound to each other in a way that make moral atomism and absolute decisional autonomy unrealistic and undesirable goals for both parties. Moreover, the philosophical atomism on which such a notion is based is of dubious viability in a complex, interrelated, technologically driven society like our own.[13]

The patient autonomy model does not give sufficient attention to the impact of disease on the patient's capacities for autonomy. We agree with Cassell that medicine should restore patient autonomy,[14] but one cannot assume that autonomy is fully restorable or preservable in cases of serious illness. Bradley formulates a telling objection to the position of Veatch, one of the most prominent ethicists arguing for the patient autonomy model. As Bradley says, "Veatch argues that the relationship between patient and doctor is an equal one, ignoring

... the fact of illness which places the patient in a potentially vulnerable relationship with his physician. . . . Based as it is on a wrong assumption, this model must be rejected when applied to the traditional doctor-patient relationship."[15]

Even the briefest experience with illness shows that ill persons often can become so anxious, guilty, angry, fearful, or hostile that they make judgments they would not make in calmer times. Patients become preoccupied with their diseases and their bodies,[16] and may see their bodies as objects that failed them. Patients are forced to reassess their values and goals. These primary characteristics of illness alter personal wholeness to a profound degree. They also change some of our assumptions about the operation of personal autonomy in the one who is ill.[17]

Healing as a moral component of the physician-patient relationship is not given sufficient weight in the autonomy model. The physician's task goes beyond the prevention of harm. It includes restoration or improvement of biological function. If health is in any degree a value of the body as a biological organism, then the physician has some obligation to work toward this good, which is intrinsic to medicine. This is the case even when the patient, in the presence of life-threatening illness, may deny or reject health. In this view both physician and patient are obliged to work toward restoration of the good of the body, which is health. We have structured elsewhere the hierarchical relationship of this good and the good of self-determination when they are in conflict in, and between, patient and doctor.[18]

Distinguished ethicists such as Childress recognize the realities of these conflicts between autonomy and paternalism. They prefer to err, if they must, on the side of autonomy on what we consider erroneous metaethical grounds, namely that rights take precedence over goods. The central point or difference in our own position is that there are better arguments, in particular instances, for the ascendancy of goods over rights.

It is, of course, increasingly true that patients with chronic, unremitting, disabling disorders, such as degenerative disorders of the nervous system, incurable neoplasms, or intractable pain, may wish to assert their right to an autonomous decision to discontinue treatment or to die. But, most often, life and health are still primary values most patients will assert over their moral and legal rights of autonomous refusal of medical care. The average patient usually assumes, too, that his or her health is still the physician's primary value as a physician. There is real danger of harm to the patient if doctor and patient misunderstand each other on this point.

Patient autonomy models often have their origins in the civil and human rights movement rather than in an ontology of relations specific to medicine and healing. Few would disavow the positive gains effected by the political struggle for human rights. But it does not follow that the adversarial presumptions of the rights movement are transferable, without modification, to the debate about the locus of medical decision making. The image of doctors as adversaries, sinister in their conspiracy against patients, is a colorful but overplayed metaphor. It stimulates scrutiny of the abuses of power than can, and all too often do, characterize medical decisions. Nonetheless, there are still physicians of character motivated by an ethics of compassion and commitment that transcends post-Enlightenment, rights-based ethical theories.[19]

Philosophical Critique of Autonomy

Our objections to autonomy as an absolute principle in medical decision making, or as a replacement for beneficence when these two principles are seemingly in conflict, need a more formal analysis than the foregoing. We find autonomy wanting in three dimensions—the contextual, the existential, and the conceptual.

Contextual Limitations

The autonomy model may not apply in some contexts of medical treatment. For example, paternalism may be appropriate when treating the aged and senile who are referred from nursing homes for urinary tract infections.[20] In such cases physicians may have an obligation to disregard the patient's wishes until they are convinced that the patient is competent. This is an example of "weak" paternalism, different in moral quality from "strong" paternalism, in which the objections of a competent patient are overruled, or in which deception is practiced to manipulate a decision.

Physicians may therefore act over the objections of patients, to preserve life or prevent serious harm, when patients are senile, confused, depressed, or otherwise incapacitated in their abilities to make autonomous judgments. The same holds for emergency room treatment. Here the uncertain prognosis, the need for an unambiguous decision, and the probability that the patient—if fully competent—would want to be treated would militate against unrestrained adherence to the patient's expressed wishes. The same may apply to hasty requests not to be resuscitated when clinical outcomes are still in doubt. On the other hand, when the clinical context is clearer and less urgent, and the patient's competence certain, autonomy can and should be given primacy.

Weak paternalism may be appropriate when treating children, in whom competence is difficult to judge or is genuinely in doubt. We may presume that, were they autonomous, children would choose to be treated—provided there is sufficient benefit to be gained from treatment. This is true, too, with therapeutic research in children. Parents may act for the good of the child in the absence of the child's consent. The context—the calculus of benefits and burdens of the experimental procedure—will determine the moral acceptability of the research. This would not be the case with nontherapeutic research that would expose a child to risk without the chance of benefit. One cannot under any doctrine of paternalism—weak or strong—presume or impose altruism on the part of another.

The clinical context may change day by day, hour by hour, even in the same patient, and with this change the moral defensibility of any act of paternalism is likewise altered.[21] Senile patients may wax and wane in competence. Acutely and desperately ill patients with severe trauma and burns may vacillate in their desire to live. While the decision to treat may be very difficult, the presumption to treat is often morally defensible if there is appreciable probability of a successful outcome. What constitutes "success" under such circumstances may be debatable, but overly hasty decisions not to treat (out of deference to the principle of autonomy) may be more damaging to the patient's ultimate best interests than some degree of paternalism.

This "variability of context" is, therefore, an important moral limitation on autonomy. It demands careful assessment in each case, even while we remain sensitive to the moral obligation to respect patient autonomy. Engelhardt also takes note of this variability and concludes that it is the product of rational disagreements about the risk-benefit calculus.[22] In his view, the variability rests on the relativity of subjective values of the interpreting parties and not on the objective difference in contexts, as we have argued.

Irrespective of its origins, context variability raises questions about any model of patient autonomy. It also underscores the need for some ranking of goods in medicine if we are to chose one ethical model over others or one moral choice over others. Any mode of clinical decision making, by virtue of the fact that it is *clinical,* must take into account the particularities and uniqueness of each human being's experience of illness.

Existential Limitations: The Fact of Illness

The effects of illness and disease on personal autonomy limit self-determination to variable degrees. That is why so many physicians report that patients really want them to make the decisions.[23] In this view autonomy ought not, therefore, be taken as a starting point or absolute ordering principle in medicine. Rather, it should be seen as part of the goal of treatment, one of the goods of the patient, to be promoted but not to the total exclusion of all other goods.

If we take the impact of illness and disease seriously, we must modify the autonomy model. That model has four features: self-direction, establishing a life plan, deliberating about applying a life plan (reasoning and information), and acting on the basis of such deliberations.[24]

Becoming "sick" can modify each of these features. To "be" sick is to be subject to the pathophysiological effects of illness, pain, and fear, and to the special professional and institutional environment in which decisions occur. Self-direction is marred by the way disease may disrupt the unity of the self, ego, and body. Life plans are threatened by the finitude of human life revealed in illness. Deliberation and application are impeded by the distractions of pain and fear, or by the process of institutionalization. The extent to which the operations of autonomy can be impeded by becoming and being a patient is impressive.

Of course, the autonomy of most patients is only mildly incapacitated by disease. We must not, therefore, use autonomy limitation as an excuse for all sorts of paternalism. On the whole, patients' choices can and should be accepted. On the other hand, people who are incapacitated by disease or trauma should not be abandoned to their autonomy, that is, merely given the "facts" and asked to make a decision. This is a form of moral abandonment. The proponents of autonomy as the prime moral obligation should give more attention to the available data about the psychosocial impact of disease on personal and moral status. A Medline search in 1985 produced *eighty-six* articles directly related to the impact of disease on autonomy and life adjustments. The data strongly suggest that autonomy is limited by illness and disease, and that any model of the doctor-patient relationship must take this limitation into account. Neither of these points is sufficiently appreciated in the current ethical debates about autonomy.

One might argue that we are merely talking about varying degrees of competence, and that the problem is one of determining competence. In this view the autonomy model would remain intact since incompetent patients could be treated paternalistically without violating the principles of autonomy. Such an interpretation would, however, offend those for whom autonomy has become an absolute principle of medical ethics.

Conceptual Limitations

The autonomy model as a model is also limited. It has been constructed in dialectical opposition to the paternalistic model, but neither paternalism nor autonomy correctly describes the full range of ethical norms governing the doctor and patient. What occurs between doctor and patient has many formulations. It can be seen as restoring autonomy, safeguarding the person,[25] respecting persons,[26] healing or restoring a lost wholeness,[27] putting the patient's needs first,[28] making a right and good medical decision,[29] or acting in the best interests of the patient.[30] Each formulation ascribes a somewhat different moral tone to the physician's obligations with respect to the patient's autonomy.

What occurs between doctor and patient in nontherapeutic research is not encompassed by any of these terms. The goal here is not primarily the benefit of the experimental subject but the discovery of knowledge. Morever, the subject's autonomy is presumably not affected by illness, or he could not give consent. In nontherapeutic research, then, respect for autonomy is mandatory as a moral principle. The duty of beneficence toward the patient would be at the lowest level of sensitivity, that is, nonmaleficence. In therapeutic research, however, the good of the patient is involved, and the questions about autonomy and paternalism would be the same as those we have already raised.

The Perils of Autonomy

The autonomy argument proceeds on the assumption that one principle should prevail in every medical situation. Libertarians such as Engelhardt often underline their commitment to this single principle.[31] We will examine Engelhardt's position in detail in the next chapter.

The ruling of the California Superior Court in the case of William Bartling is consistent with Engelhardt's conclusions, yet its shows that very strict adherence to autonomy is not always the best way to respect patients as persons. Bartling was a seventy-year-old man with chronic obstructive lung disease, a long history of smoking, coronary artery disease, and (significantly, we think) severe depression. Following a needle aspirate of a lung nodule showing adenocarcinoma, he suffered a pneumothorax and required a ventilator. After months in the intensive care unit, he sought to have the respirator removed even though he understood that it most likely would lead to his death. He often vacillated in this decision. Health care providers were uncertain whether he made this decision because of his depression, because of intensive care unit psychosis, or from the standpoint of a value commitment in his own life. After Bartling died, the Superior Court of California ruled in December 1984 that competent patients may refuse life-sustaining treatment even if they are judged to be in a terminal condition or are incapacitated by coma, and even if physicians object because of ethics or conscience.[32] A similar decision was issued in the case of Elizabeth Bouvia.[33]

In such cases we would agree with Lo's assessment of the physician's ability to ascertain more clearly than the court the medical condition of the patient, which conditions were reversible or temporarily correctable (such as the patient's possible depression), and which treatments should be instituted. Lo calls this process one of protecting patients from harm while respecting their wishes since, in the end, one would not overturn a competent person's decision.[34] A physician is justified in attempting to treat a condition that, in his best judgment, contributes to the patient's incompetent state, even if in a state of dubious competence. The contributing condition must be judged reversible and treatable for this rule to apply.[35] We will discuss this further in the last section of the book.

Indeed, respecting prior wishes of competent patients is not always the best way to respect their autonomy, as Morreim holds.[36] Had Bartling, as a clearly competent person, made prior statements about his care, and had new conditions that he could not have reasonably forseen emerged, and had these conditions been clearly reversibly using a technology he had ruled out, his physicians could have proceeded to turn the tide of the reversible disease process.

There are few absolutes at the bedside. For this reason, living will legislation in some states provides for directives to physicians that are merely advisory about the patient's preference. Physicians may sometimes act against these preferences if conditions arise that may not have been foreseen by the patient. For example, patients may refuse the respirator (anticipating dying by heart failure or cancer). They come to the hospital for a biopsy and acquire the iatrogenic disease of septic shock. The physician has, in a real way, caused this disease, and since it is under certain circumstances reversible, to benefit the patient a decision requires treatment until the patient can fully comprehend the actual circumstances and reassess his or her wishes in light of those circumstances.

In this discussion the operative concepts are "judgment," "reversible conditions," "competence," "no harm," and "respect for autonomy." No one principle is absolute enough to override any other aspect of medical and ethical decision making. Instead, a constellation of considerations, values, and ethical principles is required.[37]

On the other hand, case argumentation can be misleading. It may reduce complex situations to ones capable of being resolved by single principles, what Kopelman calls the "case-method fallacy":

> Some libertarians in their enthusiasm to alter attitudes toward the need to give adequate information and to seek consent, may select for consideration *only* cases of competent people being abused by paternalists. In contrast, paternalists may wish to promote the duties of beneficence by using *only* cases where the professional is needed to help protect or intervene on behalf of patients who are incompetent or whose choices are impaired by fear, ignorance, or pressure.[38]

Many thinkers who once proposed the primacy of autonomy over paternalism have lately come to see that no single principle can predominate so absolutely in health care ethics. Among them can be counted McCullough, who, along with Wear, critically analyzes the role of autonomy and paternalism in the beneficence model of health care.[39] Childress is another thinker who has gradually changed his position on this matter. In chapter 1 we noted his preference for rights over goods, that is, for self-determination over other values and goods such as medical intervention. We will address this claim head on in the next chapter, too, precisely because it is so central. Childress, however, now holds a somewhat modified view, in keeping with the argumentation we have advanced so far:

> It is not time to repudiate autonomy unless it is wrongly conceived as the single, exclusive, or overriding principle of biomedical ethics. What is needed is a richer portrayal of several principles and their relationships. The danger of replacing one principle by another is evident when we consider the importance of both beneficence, which supports paternalism, and respect for autonomy, which limits and constrains paternalism.[40]

Although we do not agree necessarily that beneficence supports paternalism (as will become clearer in the third section of this chapter), we agree that no single principle can predominate in all cases. In fact, we regard beneficence as a shorthand for "best interests," which includes both respect for autonomy and a benefits-to-burdens calculus about the quality of a person's life. Thus, best interest conflates several important realities and is based on neither paternalism nor autonomy.

Beyond its limitations in individual medical decisions, autonomy as a dominant ethical principle in medical ethics has serious limitations in social ethics as well. These are: (1) the movement it fosters from substantive to procedural ethics; (2) the movement from concern for the common good to individual good; and (3) the erosion of the concpet of democracy itself.

From Substance to Procedure in Ethics

One very strong impetus for the trend toward autonomy is the obvious moral pluralism of our society and the possibility that physicians and others in authority may override personal belief systems. One way to guard against this kind of moral trespass is to accept the irreconcilability of moral conflicts and turn the focus on the process of decision making. Emphasis is then placed on respect for the autonomy of the parties to a clinical decision. Most of the recommendations of the multivolume reports of the President's Commission for the Study of Ethical Problems in Medicine and Biomedical and Behavioral Research place their emphasis on procedure—informed consent, anticipatory declarations of several kinds, the proper use of proxy and surrogate decision makers, and the establishment of ethics and surrogate decision makers, and the establishment of ethics committees.[41] Many of the cases that have come to the courts have turned on the question of who shall decide, under what conditions, and by what criteria. Formalization of the decision-making process is reflected also in the recommendations of the Department of Health and Human Services pertaining to the care of terminally ill, handicapped, and physically impaired infants.[42] Engelhardt has argued particularly vigorously that the function of ethics itself in a morally pluralistic society that wishes to remain peaceable must be analysis and clarification. A particular set of values, he contends, cannot be propounded for the whole community; freedom is to be protected at all costs. Ethics, therefore, must not concern itself with moral content or normative prescriptions.[43]

This neat dissection of analytical from normative ethics is illusory. Analytical ethics does, in fact, make a normative assertion, namely, that autonomy is the first principle and that it overrides all others. Engelhardt's rigorous extrapolation of the logic of autonomy to its conclusions is the strongest argument against a purely procedural ethics. Pragmatically attractive as it may be in such a morally pluralistic and democratic society as ours, procedure cannot be self-justifying. To assert freedom as ultimate means that the search for *the* good life, and *a* good life and the good society must be abandoned. We are forced to retreat into private morality for the most meaningful questions humans ask. But this retreat brings its own serious problems with it.

Moral Atomism

The retreat to private morality eventually leads to a kind of moral atomism in which each individual's moral beliefs and actions—unless they disturb the peaceable community—are unassailable. Moral debate is not only frustrating but futile, since each person is his own arbiter of the right and the good. The traditional notion of ethics as reasoned public discourse in search of the common good is discarded. The sense of community identity that derives from some consensus on what *ought* to be done and what *ought never* to be done is lost.

The overall result is a defection from what Murray calls the "affairs of the commonwealth."[44] These affairs end up in courts, decided by legal adversarial procedure and judicial opinion, which inevitably must mix moral substance with procedure. Court opinions are already deciding substantive moral issues without the accompanying moral debate requisite to ethically sound judgment, even though ethics articles and ethics witnesses are employed.

For example, is the decision to withhold elective treatment from a Down's syndrome child the private decision of its parents based on their evaluation of quality of life, or on their personal and social burden of raising a retarded child? Moral privatism of this sort challenges government intrusion and dilutes the state's "interests." Can the obligation of government to protect the rights of the weak, the vulnerable, the comatose be abrogated on the plea of moral privacy and autonomy? The *Baby Doe* case in Bloomington, Indiana, and the *Baby Jane Doe* case in Stony Brook, Long Island, illustrate this point.[45]

It is impossible to escape the burden of doing ethics since most people still want to know whether what is procedurally acceptable is also right and good. Freedom to make one's own choices must be protected, but the flight into metaethics will not eradicate the equal need to engage as a society in the pursuit of some common moral goals beyond autonomy.

Erosion of the Idea of Democracy

Perhaps the most serious consequence of the absolutization of autonomy is the limit it places on the idea of democracy itself. Democracy is reduced to a procedure for settling otherwise irreconcilable differences among citizens, but without commitment to any common set of values except the freedom of private judgment. Certainly, one measure of a democratic society is the degree of freedom it affords for divergent and contrary opinions, but those freedoms must serve common community purpose as well.

Is not one of the traditional aims of our democracy to advance the cause of community rather than its atomization? This is our inheritance from the classical and Judeo-Christian traditions. How far may this inheritance be squandered without corroding the idea of democracy itself? How logical is the separation between public and private models? Is the purpose of government only to restrain unbridled self-interest or to promote the common good? The incommensurability of some of today's conflicting moral views shows up as private values become more selfish, more crude, more intensely combative. Power becomes the maker of morals if the common moral perspective is lost and democracy itself is weakened. Is there some choice other than that between Rousseau and Khomeini?

The sociopolitical and socioethical consequences of the move to autonomy are yet to be comprehended fully. Medical ethics—as the arena of some of the sharpest ethical debates in contemporary society—is the paradigm that brings these questions to our immediate attention. Their significance transcends medical ethics. And how we resolve them will determine what kind of society we shall have.

LIMITATIONS OF THE PATERNALISM MODEL

Just as there are formidable objections to the patient autonomy model, so, too, can objections be raised to medical paternalism. The foremost objection is that a physician often cannot heal a person just by curing a disease, especially if the physician systematically ignores or disregards the patient's view. Cassell's argument that restoring function, or curing, should be a secondary aim of medicine and that medicine's primary aim is to restore autonomy has much to recommend it.[46] It is a little extreme, however, and in its own way absolutizes autonomy, as Childress has pointed out.[47]

Healing does involve restoring autonomy. For this reason Culver and Gert are correct to insist that strong paternalism always demands justification because it violates a moral rule. But Culver and Gert do not deal directly with the moral content of medicine itself. Strong paternalism is objectionable not only because it violates moral rules, but because it violates the architectonic aim of medicine, which is to heal the one who is ill. To violate a person's autonomy is not to heal, but to wound, his or her humanity.

Strong paternalism is objectionable because it violates the humanity of the patient. Rational beings are owed the freedom to decide about the conduct of their own lives. Indeed, such decisions are peculiarly human. To infringe on such a fundamental right clearly demands special justification. Medical paternalism fails because it overrides an essential element in deontological ethics at the core of medicine, that is, respect for persons. To violate the patient's autonomy is to deprive him or her of one essential component of her own good, and thus to violate medicine's promise to act for the good of the patient.

Many physicians hold that the patient's rights to autonomy should not get in the way of their medical needs—that is, medical "indications" should dominate clinical decisions. But as we shall argue, the hierarchy of patient goods may not always place medical needs in the highest position.[48] Lack of respect for such a hierarchy of values is a major cause of patient complaints about physician paternalism.

Like the autonomy model, medical paternalism can fail to distinguish contexts and their role in medical and ethical decision making. As a consequence, medical paternalism tends to universalize a stance valid in one context but not necessarily valid in another. Generalization of one experience, like "saving" one patient through paternalism, into a universal moral posture is not valid.

Perhaps the biggest failure of medical paternalism is its assumption that medical values or the medical good is the highest good, with an absolute quality that overrides other values. Or, even less justifiably, a particular physician's preferences for one treatment among several may become an absolute. Some surgeons prefer radical mastectomy, while others prefer limited resection and radiation for cancer of the breast. Some cardiologists prefer medical over surgical management in certain types of angina pectoris. Alternative procedures may lead to similar outcomes but with different risks and quality of life. Selection of one procedure over others depends as much on the patient's and the physician's values as on the scientific data. The patient, for reasons of great importance to her, may even reject the scientifically preferred therapy for one of lesser effectiveness.

Medical paternalism asserts that the physician unequivocally knows better than the patient what is "good" for her. It also subsumes all the patient's good under only one good—medical good—a point we shall develop in more detail later. Other dimensions of the good of the patient must also be considered. One of these is surely the preservation of the fundamental human good of making one's own decisions about the kind of life one wants to lead, or the risks one wants to take.

In what ways, then, is the paternalism model inadequate? We suggest three criticisms parallel to the three philosophical critiques we leveled at the autonomy model.

Contextual Limitations

Paternalism may apply in certain limited contexts, such as making decisions over the objection of a minor about what might be best for a child, but it cannot function as a universal or general principle of medicine since it assumes something fundamentally flawed: not only that professionals know what is best for all patients, but also that they may override the patient's wishes in the pursuit of what is medically indicated. Paternalism has enjoyed such a long season because physicians can readily offer examples in which their expertise saved some patient from a truly disastrous decision. An internist of our acquaintance, for example, cites a "memorable" case in which he convinced a rabbi to have a colostomy following colonic resection for cancer. The convincing took three days of vigorous debate and discussion. In telling this tale the physician appealed to the metaphysical assumption that it is better to live than to die, to live with an impairment than to die without one. In the main, persons do accept this assumption. But not always, and not everywhere. To what extent he may or may not have justifiably exhausted the rabbi's will to autonomy is impossible to say. Given the rabbi's Talmudic training, the dialectic must have been intense and the physician's "victory" not an easy one.

Existential Limitations

Not only is context a limiting factor, but the concept of paternalism itself is also limited. It is not just a matter of the fallacy of expertise. The expert does *not* always know more about what is "best" for the nonexpert. Difficulties of prognosis and the benefits-to-burdens calculus are obvious limitations. There is also no way to define clearly what is absolutely best for the patient in medical terms alone. That definition is always related to the values the patient professes, those the institution and society assume, and those the culture holds to be important. Lacking any unequivocal definition of "benefit," the physician cannot presume to define the whole of the patient's good without essential input from the patient.

Some patients reject the benefits of medical interventions simply for their own reasons. William Bartling, as we saw, in a hospital intensive care unit in California, wished to be removed from a respirator even though he understood this would lead to his death. Some hospitals or other institutions may limit the medical benefits to be given patients. For example, Catholic hospitals rule out abortions. Nursing homes may have policies that "interpret" benefit to patients to include limitations on cardiopulmonary resuscitation.

Society defines what benefits shall be given its citizens in general, and even which medical benefits may be offered. In England there are limitations on the use of dialysis for patients older than fifty-five years of age. Respirators are removed after ten days if certain patients do not respond by that time. Finally, social values are in a constant state of definition and redefinition. At the moment our social values tend to accept the medical intervention model of beneficence. Other cultures, or subcultures within our own, may accept or reject this model.

All of these considerations put limits on paternalism. They mitigate the absoluteness of benefit from medical benefits that paternalism requires.

Conceptual Limitations Model

Paternalism as a model of the physician-patient relationship is itself flawed. At the root of this limitation is the fact that authentic healing cannot take place in a paternalistic model since paternalism overrides patient choices. Personal choice is essential to the processes of reintegration which, in turn, is essential to healing. Undeniably, "cures" can often take place in a paternalistic relationship—for example, treating pneumococcal pneumonia in an elderly patient with a stroke. This would be an "effective" and *medically* indicated, but not necessarily beneficial, treatment if the patient were dying of metastatic malignancy.

The paternalistic model also fosters a certain detachment deleterious to patient "care" and it separates cures from care. The physician tends to apply the medically indicated course of action as if the patient were, indeed, the corpus upon which one practiced the medical craft. A "cure" might ensue. But the patient's most cherished value, his or her life plan, the kind of life he might wish to have, his relationship to others, might be so violated as to vitiate the medical good. Wounding outweighs healing under such circumstances.

BENEFICENCE: A MODEL FOR MEDICAL DECISIONS

If both autonomy and paternalism have deficiencies, what model of medical decisions and clinical ethics would avoid the limitations of each—and also optimize their utility in advancing the good of the patient? We believe that a reinterpretation of the principle of beneficence can achieve these ends. The remainder of this chapter details the way we think it can do so in a model that centers on beneficence. We will develop this model further in the next two chapters.

The Principle of Beneficence: Degrees of Sensitivity
to the Good of Others

Since the model we wish to propound is grounded in the notion of beneficence, we must first outline our understanding of this essential first principle of medicine and healing. Beneficence, like the good of the patient that it presumably serves, is not a univocal or simple notion. There are levels of beneficence, as Frankena points out.[49] Just how and at what level one interprets beneficence will determine the moral obligations one feels one owes patients, and also the degree of altruism one feels obliged to practice.

The most minimal level is the level of nonmaleficence, that is, the duty to do no direct harm to another. This is the level contained in the Hippocratic prescription in the *Epidemics:* "At least do no harm." This level of beneficence is expected in any civilized society. It is enjoined even in the most extreme libertarian moral philosophies.

A further step in beneficence is the duty to prevent harm to others, that is, to remove or limit the possibilities of harm. Here we move from passive nonmaleficence to a more active intervention on behalf of others. At once, even at this minimal level, the possibility of paternalism begins to appear. For example, we might readily agree that there is a duty to remove an obstacle on a railroad track that would result in derailment and thus harm to other people. But this action might conceivably deprive some passenger who at that moment wishes to die, and would prefer to do so in a railway accident for insurance benefits, of the privilege of doing so. Most people would discount such an unlikely prospect and agree that there is a positive moral obligation to remove the object in the interest of the majority of passengers who certainly do not want to die in this way.

But what about protecting people against accidents by enforcing laws to "buckle up," to wear helmets, or to use protective goggles at work? This view of beneficence requires a more direct limitation of autonomy. While libertarians might resist this degree of paternalism, society seems to be giving certain measures such as these a sanction on the basis of harm to others. The economic costs and disability incurred by society overrule those who would elect to ignore safety requirements.

One, however, can go further and, out of the principle of preventing harm, make the growing of tobacco or the preparation of distilled liquors illegal. Here the intervention, while indirect so far as the one injured goes, is nonetheless significant for smokers and tobacco growers. Freedom and autonomy conflict with beneficence in this case in a way our society does not at this point countenance. Conceivably, it might sanction such measures at some time in the future. To do so is to raise the interpretation of beneficence to a higher degree than simple nonmaleficence.

To move still further along this scale of intervention is to interpret the duty of beneficence as binding even when it causes discomfort, risk, or pain to the benefactor. Law does not require anyone to risk life, limb, or even an inconvenience, even to save the life of another. But in medical encounters traditionally, some degree of effacement of personal self-interest has always been understood as a physician's duty. One need think only of the expectation that physicians will treat patients with contagious diseases (acquired immunodeficiency syndrome [AIDS] is a current case in point) and the scorn heaped on physicians who desert their posts in time of disaster or an epidemic. Camus' Rieux is an exemplary physician precisely because he did not desert the people of Oran, even though he might have claimed the privilege since his wife was ill elsewhere in a sanatorium.

This level of beneficence is implicit in that "higher degree of self-effacement" that Cushing terms the "common devotion" of the medical profession. It is admittedly a degree of beneficence above that expected by law or the mores of other activities such as business or relationships with neighbors or professional colleagues. It is a level, we could submit, that is essential to medicine as a moral enterprise. Without some degree of self-effacement, medicine ceases to be a profession in any traditional sense of that term and becomes only a trade or craft.

On the other hand, the degree of self-effacement expected is not the heroic or sacrificial kind. It does not require the dedication of a Mother Teresa, Albert Schweitzer, or Saint Francis. In them we move beyond duty—at least in secular terms—to supererogation, to obligations one may feel out of religious or other altruistic motives. We enter here the realm of "agapeistic" ethics—some grounded in love and charity for others.[50]

We would argue that beneficence in medical transactions should include some degree of effacement of the physician's self-interest in the interests of his or her patient. Just how much effacement is required cannot be defined in any absolute way. Many physicians today think this degree of beneficence is questionable and even objectionable. Physicians are asserting their "rights" to recreation, family life, social activity, time off, freedom to choose to treat only those who pay, to strike, and to work for investor-owned institutions. These may not be overtly unethical practices, but they are often at the moral margin where self-effacement would dictate some limit on the physician's personal interests or privileges.

For the purposes of the model we wish to advance, we will argue that the fact of illness, what it does to the sick person, and the kind of special relationship it entails with the physician dictate a degree of beneficence that goes beyond passive nonmaleficence. It includes, in our view, some obligation to act in the patient's interest even at some cost to the comfort, power, prestige, or fiscal benefit of the physician.

Objections to Beneficence

Besides the autonomy objection to beneficence we have already covered, three additional objections can be broadly formulated. The first we call the *interventionist objection,* the second identifies paternalism and beneficence, and the third we call the *social duties argument.*

The Interventionist Argument

The first objection to the beneficence model can be formulated as follows. The beneficence model is developed from too restricted a view of the doctor-patient relationship and of health care in general. From a social perspective, health care practice and its theory can be characterized as interventionist, highly technical, and intensely personal.[51] All of these characterizations influence the nature of the doctor-patient relationship; the beneficence model seems to neglect the social dimension of medical care.

In this view beneficence is anachronistic because it is rooted in a time when physicians had much less power than today; having little ability to keep patients alive in the face of serious illness in the past, they simply gave what treatment they could until the patient died or got better. No one questioned the ethics of giving every patient the maximum possible treatment because, in any case, the "maximum" did not appreciably alter the outcome.

But, the argument continues, a major change has taken place in the power of medicine. Technology permits physicians to keep people alive when even the possibility of ever regaining sentient life is remote or nonexistent. Other interventions, undreamed of even forty years ago, are now commonplace: from renal dialysis to cardiac transplantation, from cardiopulmonary resuscitation to gene therapy or total renal replacement. Given the power of medicine and its impact on the individual, a paternalistic, interventionist ethic is inadequate; decisions about care must be based on the patient's expressed wishes. Hence, the autonomy model is better suited than the beneficence model to today's health care.

It is true that modern medicine may appear to be and can be used as a high-technology, interventionist monolith, but these features are less the result of the beneficence model than of the complex instrumentation of medical technology, and the institutions and organization required to deliver it. To be sure, these factors, accentuated by value-free attitudes and medical entrepreneurship, can overpower the physician as well. The objection fails because these "evils" are not an intrinsic part of the beneficence model. They are, in fact, as inimical to that model as they are to the autonomy model.

But this objection to beneficence has a stronger form than its interventionist quality. It is also based on changes in the social fabric and the alterations they induce in the forms of medical practice. On this point Siegler wryly describes the "ages" of medicine as follows: He dubs the time from Hippocrates to 1965 the "age of paternalism." This period was superceded by the "age of autonomy," which lasted until October 1, 1983, when the "age of bureaucratic parsimony" began with the inauguration of diagnostic-related groups for Medicare and Medicaid patients. As Siegler points out in the previous two ages, the patient's good was the principal concern for physicians. In the age of paternalism, good was defined as the patient's best medical interest. In the age of autonomy, the goods sought were the patient's freedom and right of self-determination. In the age of bureaucratic parsimony, however, the good of the patient will have to be balanced against other goods, such as the needs of the hospital, the needs of its employees (including physicians), and the needs of society.[52]

The objection to beneficence, which of course is *not* Siegler's thesis, is that the ages of medicine have passed it by. A new calling is proposed for physicians, requiring them to be gatekeepers of health care institutions, the new watchdogs of social policy and society's resources.

At the root of the second objection to beneficence is its identification with paternalism, coupled with an emphasis on autonomy. In this view, every form of acting for the good of another is suspect. Even Siegler's comment above that the best interests of patients during the age of autonomy was to preserve their self-determination still seems, to critics, to smack of paternalism. Looking out for others somehow is seen as a violation of their autonomy.

Paternalism and Beneficence Identified

Beneficence and paternalism are often seen as intrinsically identical. An effort by one of us to formulate broader conceptions of freedom than the often narrowly construed notion of autonomy is a good example.[53] It was regarded by Kvale, a geriatric specialist, as "nothing more than a thinly veiled attempt to reinstitute paternalism."[54]

It is true, of course, that many famous court cases have involved the fight to assert important patient rights. They moved health care from the "paternalistic age" to the "autonomy age." Most of these cases involved the sometimes very harmful demands of high-technology, interventionist medicine. Examples in point are using or withdrawing the respirator from Karen Ann Quinlan, and treating Joseph Saikewicz, an older mentally retarded patient with leukemia. Other examples are those of William Bartling and Elizabeth Bouvia, already mentioned, and the indictment for murder of Drs. Robert Nejdl and Neil Barber, who withdrew a respirator from a comatose man after surgery and later removed the patient's nasogastric feeding tube and intravenous lines. More recently the New Jersey Supreme Court, concerning *In the matter of Claire C. Conroy,* considered the issue of withdrawing the nasogastric feeding tube, this time from a weak, debilitated, and senile woman who was not at the time dying.[55] These cases are now part of the growing heritage of medical ethics. They have led to important distinctions about care, about our duties toward the dying and the incapacitated, and about the validity of quality-of-life judgments.

None of these considerations, however, can be seen as an objection to the beneficence model. It might be tempting to think that these cases give precedence to patient wishes or presumed wishes over physician paternalism, but that is not so. Instead, they emphasize patient wishes (or those of guardians speaking on behalf of patients) as a means for protecting the patient's best interests. This is a critical point. While autonomy is not a clear winner in these cases, neither is paternalism. Rather, the best interests of the patients are intimately linked with their preferences. From these are derived our primary duties toward them. It is not simply a matter of negotiating a number of distinct but relative values, as libertarians would have it. Rather, axioms or "tests" (to use the New Jersey Supreme Court language) guide the decision to be made, under the general principle of beneficence.

The Social Duties Argument

The social duties argument is directed against the emphasis of beneficence models on the primary obligation of the physician toward his or her individual patients. Beneficence, it is objected, is too preoccupied with the patient, to the exclusion of social duties. Thus, the physician concerned about a diabetic and pregnant patient on Medicaid would be concerned primariy with her good and her best interests, not with those of society or even of other similarly situated patients.

Against this primary patient-orientation of beneficence it is held that the doctor and the patient are actually social beings, within the context of a social relationship whose characteristics are predominantly social. Hence, what should be of primary ethical concern are the issues of power, the social nature of the profession, and the role-specific obligations and duties that bind both doctor and patient.[56] Most medical practices are allied with hospitals and other health care institutions, with concomitant ease of access to high-technology intervention. There are few truly "solo" practices in the United States today. In addition, the trend toward medical entrepreneurship leads physicians and other health care professionals such as nurses and social workers to establish cooperatives, joint ventures, and corporations.[57] These changes have altered the traditional autonomy of the physician in private practice, so that, in addition to negotiation with the patient, the physician must also be more aware of the constraints placed on his or her judgments by hospitals, partners in practice, and other health provisions.[58]

Further, it is argued that in an age of cost containment, the physician must now assume a new social duty, that of gatekeeper, controlling access to expensive high-technology care. In health maintenance organizations (HMOs) the physician is required to constrain tests, treatments, consultations, and hospitalizations. If a physician were always to act in the best interests of the patient, then, she might bankrupt an HMO. In preferred provider organizations physicians are given even more concrete incentives to control costs. They may, in some plans, receive a bonus based on the amount of money the organization saves in a year. The AMA Judicial Council has rejected this scheme as dangerous and unethical.

These examples clearly indicate a set of social expectations that move beyond more traditional notions of the doctor's primary obligation to his or her patient. Most certainly at risk in these new obligations are the connotations of beneficence developed thus far in this book.

An answer to this objection is based not on the denial of social obligations to medicine but on the deleterious effects of absolutizing either social or individual obligations. We do recognize the changes that have been brought about by medical technology. The medical practitioner must now negotiate with many different health professionals from many different subspecialties about her care and treatment plan. As a consequence, uncritical appeals to traditional statements about the doctor-patient relationship, however uplifting, can become empty rhetoric. The fact of social change in medical practice is too evident to ignore in modern theories of medicine.

This is not to say that a seminal work by Lain-Entralgo on the doctor-patient relationship is suddenly made invalid.[59] Rather, it is to admit, as he himself did, that the character of the doctor-patient relationship changes over time. Yet its continual object is to provide for the best interests of the patient and, thereby, of society. Our own previous work on the philosophy of medicine was predicated upon a search through the history of Western medicine for perduring, axiomatic values in medicine. We think we have discovered some axioms we interpret as norms; if violated, these norms vitiate the very character of the doctor-patient relationship itself as a healing encounter. But the norms themselves must always function with regard to social context.[60]

Merely to discover that beneficence is a persisting value throughout the history of the doctor-patient relationship is not sufficient, given the actual changes in modern medicine and the pressures to change. It must also be defended, as we attempt to do in this book.

Perhaps the most immediate challenges to beneficence as the primary principle in medicine come at present from obligations physicians might have to society or to a health organization to control costs. There is no doubt that, under certain circumstances, denying a patient access to care for economic reasons directly violates the notion of beneficence.

Veatch proposes that physicians have social obligations in justice from which they are exempted in order to care for individuals. In his draft medico-ethical covenant, Veatch proposes that

> individual practitioners shall be exempt from the general moral requirements of the principles of justice, including their impact on health care planning and cost-containment, insofar as they are committed to patients in ongoing lay-professional relationships. However, the needs of one's own patients shall be taken into account in deciding how to allocate one's professional time among patients in need, and the extreme needs of nonpatients shall be taken into account in deciding whether to sacrifice temporarily the marginal welfare of one's patient in order to meet the desperate need of a nonpatient.[61]

Veatch's proposal still places primary stress on the obligation to individual patients. In this his viewpoint is like ours. While his is a creative effort to deal with the doctor's dilemma, it strikes us as odd to consider the relationship with the patient as an exemption from justice rather than an expression of it.[62] Our resolution follows somewhat different lines. We hold that the primary duty of the physician is to act in the best interests of his or her patient. This action must proceed at the bedside with regard for efficiency and moderation in health care costs. This is best accomplished by the practice of diagnostic elegance and therapeutic parsimony. Here efficiency and cost moderation do not clash with the direct benefit to the patient because they would not be used primarily to cut costs. Instead, tests would not be ordered for the sole purpose of protecting the physician or the hospital from lawsuits;[63] they would not be ordered unless they were demonstrably useful in making a diagnosis. Treatments without demonstrable effect on the routine history of the disease would be avoided.

Finally, none of the above argument denies the duty of physicians to cooperate or, indeed, lead in a national discussion of the proper allocation of health care. All health care professionals share this duty, as do the hospitals and institutions in which they practice. In particular, it is important that the traditional duty of physicians to treat all patients regardless of their ability to pay be preserved and expanded to society as a whole.[64] Not many Americans would disagree with the president's commission report, *Securing Access to Health Care,* which states, "Society has an ethical obligation to ensure equitable access to health care for all."[65]

With this discussion of beneficence in hand, let us turn to the model we feel most closely exemplifies the duties physicians owe patients.

Major Features of the Beneficence Model

Given the shortcomings we have pointed out in both the patient autonomy and the medical paternalism models, is there an alternative that does not reduce to one or the other? We suggest there is, though we appreciate that the complexity of the physician-patient relationship can never be adequately described in a single model. Our purpose in sketching the beneficence model is to circumvent the substantial problems with the models we have already mentioned. We do not claim that the physician-patient relationship is fully defined by this model either. The six major features of the beneficence model are described below.

The Aim of Medicine Is Beneficent

Medicine as a human activity is of necessity a form of beneficence. It is a response to the need and plea of a sick person for help, without which the patient might die or suffer unnecessary pain or disability. The obligation to help the sick is a general one involving humans, even those who are not professed healers. It is grounded in the claim that comes from the vulnerability and suffering of a fellow human. One is impelled, even by the lesser degrees of beneficence, not to harm and, in fact, to ease suffering.

When one is a professed healer, one possesses knowledge and skill that society has permitted one to acquire precisely because they can benefit others. One also promises to help and to act on behalf of the good of the patient when one offers oneself to another as a healer. Further, without the special knowledge the healer has acquired, others would suffer, so in a sense all the sick have some claim on all healers.[66]

Beneficence is a prime requirement for medicine and has three specific obligations. First, the patient's problems and needs are the physician's primary concern, taking precedence, except in the rarest circumstances, over all other concerns. Second, harm must be avoided because the physician cannot fulfill the promise of helping if he or she intentionally harms the patient for any reason. Third, both autonomy and paternalism are superseded by the obligation to act beneficently; that is to say, the choice of whether one acts to foster autonomy or instead acts paternalistically should be based on what most benefits the patient and not on the intellectual convictions or emotional impulses of the physician.

Primacy of the Existential Condition of the Patient

The second feature of the beneficence model is the primacy of the existential condition of the patient rather than of traditional professional codes. A good example can be found in Siegler's criteria for deciding the limits of autonomy to be accepted by a physician treating a seriously ill patient.[67] These criteria include the patient's ability to make rational choices about care; the nature and past values of the patient; the age of the patient; the nature of the illness; the values of the physician who must make a choice in the care of the patient; and the clinical setting, especially the diffusion of care. The first four items deal with the personal condition of the patient, and the last two deal with the health care professional and environment. Presumably, Siegler does not mean that age should be considered an independent variable in making decisions, but rather, as his subsequent writings would suggest, that age is a valuable marker of the condition of the patient.

No Automatic Ranking of Values

Both the patient autonomy model and the medical paternalism model emphasize single values that are always to be preferred. For example, the patient's right to autonomy is always to be preferred over other values in the patient autonomy model. In the paternalism model each patient must be treated as if he or she did not know what is best. By contrast, in the beneficent model, clinical values are not ranked in any preset hierarchy. Each patient must be handled individually not only for the medical, but also for the moral, implications. No ethical stance, other than acting for the patient's best interest, is applied beforehand. This model requires that patients and physicians become able to identify, rank, discuss, and negotiate values,[68] and define the particular good of a particular patient. This is *not* to say, however, that general ethical axioms applied to more than one patient are invalid.

Consensus

The fourth feature of the beneficence model is consensus. Because there is to be no imposition of values, or decisions made in the best interest of patients without their participation, a consensus with the patient and with other members of the health care team is needed. Admittedly, a consensus model takes time and energy, but it also wards off many agonizing hours of later conflict in the course of a serious illness. In fact, one of the seductions of the autonomy and paternalism models is their comparative ease of decision making: Either the physician makes all the decisions or the patient does so. Both models abandon the trials and rewards of a mutual dialogue and exchange between doctor and patient.[69] Both also can assault the moral agency of the patient or the physician.

A consensus reached at the beginning of a patient's care cannot be assumed to continue unchanged as new developments occur. The consensus must be monitored for its continued validity. This requires a continuing dialogue between the patient and his or her medical attendants.

Prudential Moral Object

The fifth feature is a prudential moral object, that is, an attempt must be made to resolve difficult ethical quandaries by preserving as many values of both the patient and physician as possible. Ackerman has argued that this should be the goal of bioethics.[70] Whether or not one agrees entirely, it is a goal of a consensus-driven, patient-oriented approach in which prudential judgments are made on a patient-by-patient basis.

Axioms

Explicit axioms represent the sixth and last major feature of the beneficence model. Just as the physician examines each patient in light of generalized theories or categories of disease and health, his or her prudential judgment about each patient must adhere to a series of more general ethical axioms or moral rules. These are necessary to avoid the moral pitfalls of the autonomy and paternalism models, as well as those of situational ethics.

Axioms of the Beneficence Model

1. *Both doctor and patient must be free to make informed decisions and to act fully as moral agents.* The values of both doctor and patient must be respected since each is a person deserving of respect as such. Value consensus results only if each can, without coercion or deception, express his or her own values in discourse and action. Neither can impose his or her values on the other; neither can "use" the other for selfish ends; each must be free to withdraw from the relationship if value conflicts are not resolvable.[71]

2. *Physicians have the greater responsibility in the relationship because of the inherent inequality of information and power between themselves and those who are ill.* Physicians are obliged, therefore, to provide the information patients need to make genuinely informed decisions, and to use their power with due regard for the vulnerability and exploitability of the sick. These obligations are rooted in the special nature of the healing relationship. The self-imposed moral aims of the profession and the expectations of society derive their force from this fact as well.

3. *Physicians must be persons of personal moral integrity.* The physician must have the capacity to make prudential judgments that factor in the particulars of each case, the general features of the disease, and general moral principles. Ultimately, the good of the patient depends as much on the physician's character as on his or her capacity to make these judgments and the extent to which the physician can be trusted to keep the good of the patient as her primary aim.[72] In a morally pluralistic society, there is a tendency to downplay moral character in the education of the physician. However, there are qualities of moral judgment that should apply to all physicians, and for this they will need to be educated. As Aristotle noted, "It is impossible, or not easy, to do noble acts without the proper equipment."[73] Skill in making ethical judgments must

be taught in medical schools.[74] Yet skills without moral integrity will not suffice in those moments when no one is there to watch and the good of the patient hangs on the moral integrity of the physician.

4. *Physicians must respect and comprehend moral ambiguity yet not abandon the search for what is right and good in each decision.* By training and disposition physicians are inclined to diagnostic closure and problem resolution. They are dismayed when there is no single "right" answer to a moral dilemma. Yet, in the beneficence model this may often be the case since the good is defined by principles and individuals in their life contexts without standardized formulae. Physicians must avoid the pitfalls so aptly described by MacIntyre: "It is a central feature of contemporary moral debates that they are unsettleable and interminable. . . . because no argument can be carried through to a victorious conclusion, argument characteristically gives way to the mere and increasingly shrill battle of assertion with counter-assertion."[75] No matter how frustrating moral "debates" may be, the physician still must make moral decisions with, and for, his or her patients. It is incumbent upon him, therefore, to learn how to deal with the reality of moral ambiguity. He has not the scholar's luxury of "on the one hand" and "on the other hand." He just acts, and to act is to choose among alternatives—moral as well as technical.

CONCLUSION

The values of patient welfare and patient autonomy—which translate into the corresonding moral duties of beneficence and respect for persons—may come into conflict with each other. In our view, however, these duties cannot remain in conflict if medicine is to achieve its goal of healing.

But healing, as we define it, is a form of assistance in making the patient whole again by working through his or her body. If the values of patient welfare and patient autonomy remain in conflict, then authentic healing cannot take place. A physician, therefore, must become both a moderate autonomist and a moderate welfarist. This can be accomplished in a beneficence model such as the one we suggest.

Another way of arriving at this position is to consider the principle of respect for persons. This principle leads to at least two moral duties. The first is to respect the self-determination or autonomy of others. The second, often-neglected duty is to help restore that autonomy or help establish it when it is absent. Looked at in this way, beneficence is seen to be a direct consequence of a fundamental moral principle and the guiding duty of medicine. If this is true, then the autonomy model is necessarily incomplete. So, too, is the paternalistic model.

Beneficence is the principle that prompts physicians to cite their moral commitments and personal support for patients beyond just respecting their rights. It is beneficence, not authoritarianism, as he incorrectly supposed, that prompted Ingelfinger to argue that doctors must recommend a course of action. Most just lay out alternatives and abandon patients.[76] It is beneficence, too, not just respect for autonomy that, properly protects patients' rights. It is the primary duty of beneficence, and not paternalism, that has historically been the guiding norm of medicine.

To be sure, beneficence can be and has been subverted into paternalism. But if our task is "proposing revised values," as Callahan asserts,[77] then it is important to focus on the virtue of benevolence (or the principle of beneficence) rather than the rule of autonomy. This virtue is consistent with the ethical tradition of persons united in community. This is a tradition more in keeping with the ethical roots of medicine than one that stresses autonomous individualism.

In the next two chapters, we will deal with additional objections to the beneficence model. In this way we hope to further refine its meaning.

3

Why Good Rather than Rights?

This chapter's purpose is to justify our position that an emphasis on the good of the patient is essential today to balance the current overemphasis on patient autonomy propounded by some ethicists, patients, and physicians. While we accept the present emphasis on autonomy as a justifiable reaction to medicine's historical paternalism, we wish to further elaborate the perils of unrestrained autonomy as well. To this end we present first the metaphysical substratum of the beneficence-autonomy conflict in two opposing ethical theories. Then we propose a relationship theory of health as the good in medicine. Finally, we develop the theory against the backdrop of autonomy and paternalism. This theory forms the basis for subsequent chapters and explains why refusal of treatment is a relative, rather than an absolute, moral right.[1]

THE METAPHYSICAL SUBSTRATUM

In the last chapter we showed how recent history has led to a critique of paternalism in medicine, but only more recently to a critique of autonomy. We have argued elsewhere that a philosophy of medicine is essential to any effective consideration of this question.[2] Without it, we are reduced to simple assertion and counterassertion, which is not only frustrating but counterproductive. A philosophy or theory of medicine implies at least a coherent structure of ideas that can be critically and formally examined. There can be few answers unless some negotiation of positions takes place. And there are good reasons for claiming that negotiation is critical to the future of medicine. Physicians understandably balk at their reduction to mere functionaries of patient wishes, just as patients now balk at their reduction to infantile dependency on physicians.

We consider the clear and present danger of the times to be this: that in demonstrating the rightness of their cause against paternalism, patients, lawyers, judges, and ethicists may discard the most important value of medicine—acting for the good of the patient, which we have argued elsewhere is an inherent function of clinical judgment.[3]

At least in part, the overemphasis on patient autonomy stems from two competing systems of ethics, both claiming social acceptance and medical relevance. The first, which we arbitrarily call system A, is largely deductive. It argues to conclusions from general ethical principles. In this process it takes only momentary cognizance of realities and the peculiarities of different situations, since the general principle is conceived to be a good in all instances. System A has tended to be Kantian, that is, a system that proposes *respect for persons* as the highest moral principle or good. In keeping with the spirit of the Enlightenment in which the system was nurtured, it has also tended to be individualistic, assuming that respect for persons requires respect for the rights and entitlements of individuals.

This system of ethics tended to dominate the early years of Anglo-American medical ethics (1960–80). One might easily predict where its reasoning would lead. Consider, for example, Veatch's early claim that physicians should not be part of decisions patients make when they are dying because they are not particularly well versed in ethics.[4] The reasoning for this claim might be as follows:

- One must respect persons.
- But persons are self-determining.
- Therefore one must respect self-determination.
- Self-determination about one's death is of utmost importance.
- But physicians are not part of the process of self-determination about death.
- Hence physicians should not be involved in decisions about death made by dying patients.

An earlier example of system A reasoning in medical ethics was Ramsey's argument, in his influential book *The Patient as Person,* that children cannot consent to, and therefore cannot participate in, research on experimental therapies on the grounds of respect for persons and autonomy.[5] The argumentation Ramsey follows rests on deductive reasoning. It goes like this:

- Respect for persons demands consent for the protection of autonomy.
- Children cannot consent because they are minors.
- Further, their consent would be set in the context of coercion by parents and health care providers and researchers, since they could not understand the consequences of their decision nor the complexities of the scientific research to be conducted.
- Hence they should not be asked to participate in such research.

A more recent example of system A thinking, one that we saw in chapter 1, is Childress' argument that paternalism is a prima facie wrong not because of its consequences or because it violates the moral rules, as Culver and Gert claim,[6] but because it violates the very principle of respect for persons.[7] As we saw, Childress does not think that what is remarkable (wrong) about paternalism is the fact that it overrides a moral rule. Rather, it violates the right to self-determination (autonomy). It is therefore always wrong. It is always wrong because it abuses the principle of respect for persons.

This kind of reasoning tends to gloss over medical realities. In the Veatch example the intimate relation between a physician and a dying patient, especially the former's role as the dying patient's advocate,[8] is neglected in favor of the general ethical principle of patient autonomy. In like fashion, Ramsey's argument ignores the fact that some research involving experimental therapy with children is required because childrens' responses to illness and medication are different from those of adults. Also, the most promising therapies, especially in cancer, often turn out to be experimental therapies. Some effective drugs are available only in experimental protocols.

System B reasoning stresses social responsibility and social good over the rights of individuals. Unlike system A, its arguments often reason from social consequences back to arguments for conduct. System B may also argue deductively from principles. If it takes this form, however, the principle is utilitarian (maximize the good) rather than respect for persons, as in system A. System B is often perceived, from the narrow window of recent ethical theory, to be a form either of repudiated utilitarianism, in which one seeks the greatest good for the greatest number, or of antiquated natural law theory.

Thus, McCormick's argument against Ramsey's earlier views about research on children takes the position that children, as members of society, owe society a responsibility to participate in research.[9] McCormick's position is clearly more dependent on the place of a child in the family of human beings than is Ramsey's. Ramsey's starting point is individualistic autonomy, while McCormick's is the person in society, a sort of modified natural law ethical position. McCormick then reasons that, as we are social beings with responsibilities to others, it is good for parents and physicians to enter children on research protocols because it teaches the child (if he or she is old enough) that there are obligations to help others.

In an apparent modification of his earlier deontological position, Ramsey later argued in favor of a "medical indications policy" for treatment of the dying on the grounds that a patient's right to refuse treatment is a relative right—relative, that is, to social duties and responsibilities as a member of a community.[10] Hence, one must accept certain obligatory medically indicated treatments. Ramsey argues that a patient may not refuse life-sustaining treatment because, if it is medically indicated, the patient must accept it on the grounds of duties to the community. Ramsey proposes that a person does not have an absolute right to refuse treatment. This position is surely a minority view among ethicists today. We will examine the limitation on the right to refuse treatment later in this chapter.

Concerned about the social duties of physicians in his earlier thinking (for example, with respect to their right to strike[11]), Veatch has developed a nonconsequentialist theory of social duties based on a covenant model of the doctor-patient relation.[12] According to this model physicians have primary social obligations. However, society, through the covenant with individual patients, exempts physicians from their social duties so they can care for individuals. Greater needs can nonetheless override this covenant. An example might be a physician who, while caring for a patient at a routine office checkup, is summoned to the street to help two accident victims. The duty to lend assistance in this type of social emergency is a primary duty, and easily outweighs the duty to the individual patient. The difficulty with this model and its examples is that it so emphasizes social obligations that it seems to view obligations to individual patients as an exemption from, rather than an expression of, justice.[13]

The dialectic between systems A and B is at root a metaphysical one. System A stresses individual rights, and system B stresses social goods. As Childress has perceptively recognized, there is a metaphysical option—one chooses either rights or goods.[14] Recently, however, all the emphasis and development have been on a theory of rights. What is urgently needed now is an equal development of a theory of goods in medicine that is independent of utilitarian or traditional natural law theory, one that can hold its own with a theory of rights. Our proposal should be seen as a first step in this regard.

A THEORY OF RELATIONAL GOOD

If our perception of the current dialectic is correct, then what is needed is a stronger theory of the good in medicine. We would argue that health functions in medicine as a *relational good,* that is, as a prominent value for both patient and physician in relation to one another. By relational good, therefore, we mean a good that arises within a human relationship. By definition, it cannot be an absolute good to which one must adhere in any event. Taking this point of view means that we cannot agree entirely with Ramsey's medical indications policy, although we do agree with him that the right to refuse treatment is not an absolute right. Ramsey bases his argument on the duties a person has to society and to other members of the human race. This duty requires that treatments to save one's life, if medically indicated, must be accepted.

Our view of the relational good by contrast, does not obligate individuals to accept one or another form of treatment. Rather, the relative importance of the right to refuse treatment arises from the way "health as a value" functions within the doctor-patient relationship, and from the mutual commitments each has made to the other. Different weights are also brought to bear on health from other values the patient cherishes, a point that will be amplified later in this book.

Ramsey most forcefully developed his medical indications policy in cases involving infants. He wished to preserve the presumption to treat defective newborns and infants. Since the infant cannot express its wishes, the medically indicated course of action must be followed. In these cases a relational good as we have defined it is not possible. We must ground our judgment of beneficence on the assumption that, if they could speak, infant patients would want us to act in their best interest. In the absence of other preferred wishes, then, one must choose the medically indicated course of action. On this point we do agree with Ramsey. Medical indications guide a proper course of action that will most likely benefit the patient.

With incompetent or never-competent patients, the relational good involves the surrogate or proxy decision maker. Under the following specified conditions, the surrogate or proxy may reject "medically indicated treatments": (1) evidence that the patient would have wanted to reject treatment as provided in an anticipatory declaration of some kind (for example, an advance directive or living will); (2) absence of conflict of interest on the part of the proxy; (3) a competent proxy; and (4) absence of past serious emotional or psychological conflicts between proxy and patient that might impel the proxy to "get even" by undertreatment or assuage guilt by overtreatment.

Another aspect of relational good is the conformity or nonconformity of the decision of a competent patient or proxy with moral good as perceived by the physician. As a moral agent the physician cannot be expected to violate his or her own values. If the physician believes that the medically indicated treatment is indeed in the patient's best interests, and that it would be morally wrong not to treat, she should respectfully withdraw. She should first provide assurance that another physician acceptable to the patient or proxy will take over the case.

Our theory can be seen as system C, incorporating the best of systems A and B without succumbing to their weaknesses. At this point in our exploration, the distinction between systems A, B, and C lies not in whether they are deductive but in the differences in their starting premises.

We hold that system C has a chance to succeed in expressing values for both patients and physicians because it is grounded in the nature of medicine itself and in the nature of human beings. It owes a great deal to Aristotle, the empiricists, and the pragmatists. It is our contention that theories based on the practice of medicine, but not limited thereto, are less likely to ignore the realities of medicine in favor of abstract ethical principle. Yet because medicine is based on health as a primary value, the values protected by ethical principles are preserved. What we propose is in reality a medical axiology—a value theory of medicine derived from the realities of the medical transaction itself.[15]

We do not offer our axiology as a foil to an already successful and more plausible theory. Rather, we offer it as a more plausible solution to the autonomy-paternalism debate than a rock-steady repetition of Kantian ethics. We also avoid absolutizing either the utilitarian or the natural law theory.

Because our human capacities are challenged to the full in society, we must learn, even as children, the consequences and limitations of making choices. Because the capacity to choose is exercised within the community, we are obliged by the rights of others and the very power of this capacity to set limits on it. Those limits include not harming others, or not violating values held in common, without reason. The power and authority of our moral beliefs, and of our ethical values, theories, and principles, derive their validity from both real-ity and the consensus of the community. That is why Nielsen and MacIntyre have so frequently and so cogently attacked deductive systems of ethics. They show that the ethical principles from which conclusions are deduced may not represent a consensus in a morally pluralistic society.[16,17]

Thus, what is most important about autonomy as a value is not that the person exercising voluntary choices is an isolated individual, but that his or her choices and autonomy are rooted in the person, who, in turn, is a member of the community. Though the choice creates an individually interpreted morality, the moral choices and values arise out of and return back to the community. The capacity to choose is the one feature that distinguishes humans from other animals precisely because it establishes a network of rights and obligations toward individuals and toward society. Thus, even autonomy is to be respected within a community context. It is also relational.

What is the object of choices, then? The object is a perceived good. The process of pursuing such goods has been called *valuing,* and goods as objects of valuing have been called *values.* We prefer the more sophisticated understand-ing of values advanced by Hartman, namely, that values are either intrinsic, extrinsic, or systemic patterns or relative weights given to properties of things or things themselves.[18] Hence, a relational theory of the good in medicine under-lines the relation of goods to human perceptions and choices, and to properties within and among things which, constantly readjusted in worth by human beings, are in continual and proportional flux.

In this way health as a good can be understood to be a value. First, it is a value because it is the aim of individuals and society. In this sense it is a nor-mative value. Second, we may understand it to be a value, a relational good, because it is the object of human and social choices. Health as a value functions in the third sense as the object of conduct and policy, not just as an end one might wish to pursue.

The implications of this theory for medicine are significant. For one thing, it means that our choice need not be limited to promoting individual good at the expense of social good of vice versa. In medicine there is a profession of the good as a tertium quid, a third reality that conflates individual and social good. Health is simultaneously an individual and a social good. To choose it is to choose both individual enhancement and social well-being. By this we do not mean to escape the difficult problems raised by the tension between individual and society. Nor do we mean that health must be defined, as it was by the World Health Organization, as a state of complete physical, mental, and social well-being. Rather, we mean that ethical systems A and B establish a false dichotomy if they present choice between individual autonomy and the greatest good of society as the only option.

Medical good is neither exclusively the good of an individual nor the good of society. The primal value in medicine is neither individual autonomy nor social well-being. It is, rather, the obligation of healers to serve the good of their patients. The ideal good of medicine, therefore, is not fully represented by eth-ical principles drawn from the deontological or utilitarian tradition. The good is a relation between doctor and patient in which healing is an object and, further, in which the ethical challenge is the moral management of the many and variegated relations that occur therein—relations between doctor and patient, intrinsic and extrinsic values, individual and social needs, personal and institutional aims, and the like.

AUTONOMY REEXAMINED

In chapter 3 we said that the beneficence model, unlike the paternalism and autonomy models, did not provide for the primacy of any one value over others except the good of the patient. No preset hierarchy other than the good of the patient is established by the assertion that one must act in the best interests of one's patients. But as we have explored the notion further in this chapter, we have seen that some preferences do occur in certain situations.

Discussions of autonomy usually center on the right of individuals to make their own decisions. Since the Enlightenment this right has been grounded in an inherent claim we all have on each other as humans. Kant argued the case for moral agency on the basis of the intrinsic dignity of the human person. He did not explicitly ground that case in human nature, but he was, implicitly at least, still in the classical and medieval tradition that did so.

If autonomy is not to be a prelogical presupposition to ethics—and it is, in fact, assuming such a position in our society—then it must be grounded in something more fundamental. We would ground it in what it means to be human, to make explicit what is implicit in Kant's deontology or moral agency. If we do so, then autonomy becomes less of an absolute principle—it is subject to limitations by some higher principle or, at least, it can be examined from the perspective of other obligations that follow from the fact of our being human.

In essence, we seek a clarification of the possible limitations on the freedom of individual choice. What might those limitations be? We would suggest several: (1) the constraints our choice places on the choice of others; (2) conflict between our choices and transcendent sources of morality, for those who accept such sources; and (3) conflicts with other goods of human beings.

One source of conflict often neglected or predetermined in the current dominance of autonomy over beneficence is the conflict between freedom of choice as a good and the good of the body. Are we free to deny the good of the body—our own and others'—in deference to the right to reject treatment? Is there not a higher good—not in the patient's perception of things, but in the natural order, an order to which the patient must at least in some sense submit?

One such order of good is the good of the body as a biological organism, one whose natural end is good function, admittedly at the service of the person or the person's goals. But can the body be only instrumental and totally submissive to whatever ends its "owner" puts it? This strikes us as yet another excessively Cartesian view of the body. Contrast this view with that of Marcel, whom we cited in our earlier book in developing our own ontology of the body for a philosophy of medicine. He has written, "I *am* my body insofar as I succeed in recognizing that this body of mine *cannot,* in the last analysis, be brought down to the level of being this object, *an* object, a something or other."[19]

We call this perception the *lived body.* Note that the lived body is formed in the community and is shaped by the community, its values, and its history. Further, the lived body is formed by the biological processes that occur as a person grows from zygote to senior citizen. Considering both the social and the biological bases of the body, then, it is difficult to agree that it is totally under the dominance of its processes. Cannot one argue that to pursue any ends, good or bad, to their fullest potential the body must be healthy? Of course, one may pursue many good human ends with a diseased or disabled body. But is it not the end of persons to seek the highest possible fulfillment of the potentialities with which they have been endowed? Is it not a violation of the good of the body to mistreat it by excesses (tobacco, alcohol, drugs, food, sloth) or to fail to repair it when an effective means of repair is available? If this is so, then it follows that there is a limitation on autonomy—for example, when it radically rejects curative and beneficent treatment that offers the genuine possibility of a return of function in whole or in part. In our view of the good of the body, each treatment would be required.

The practical question in clinical decisions is not whether or not we have a right to autonomy. We most certainly do. Rather, the question centers on the proper exercise of autonomy. Do we have a right to exercise autonomy when the decision we wish to make is not morally good? Are we free to make morally wrong decisions? Engelhardt, argues that such freedom must be guaranteed to maintain a peaceable society. In such a society, when there is no agreement on principle regarding what constitutes morally good and morally bad decision making—or in fact, what constitutes good and evil—the highest form of respect for persons is to ensure individual liberties.[20]

THE PRIMACY OF AUTONOMY

In Englehardt's godless but peaceable secular society, autonomy is required as a condition of possibility for morality. The moral principle of keeping peace by respecting autonomy makes negotiation about values in relationships possible. In this way respect for individual values is guaranteed. Mutual respect defines those persons who adhere to morality; lack of respect for persons characterizes moral outlaws.[21]

By contrast, the idea of beneficence is seen as somewhat vacuous since the good aimed at in beneficence is open to diverse cultural interpretations and individual judgments. Early in his book Englehardt views autonomy as setting the boundaries of morality while beneficence defines its content—"what is good or bad to do"—in general and specific instances. The right to autonomy in this libertarian view takes precedence over the good: "Respect of the principle of autonomy binds all persons together in the moral life. Respect of particular principles of beneficence separates communities. Respect of the general principle of beneficence reminds individuals from different moral communities of the common commitment to doing the good, even when the visions of the good diverge."[22]

Autonomy is defined, then, as a maxim: "Do not do to others that which they would not have done to them, and do for them that which one has contracted to do."[23] As the book progresses, the focus on individual autonomy becomes ascendant, and the role of beneficence as the basis of a community's or a person's articulation of values and goods drops out of Englehardt's analysis.

Indeed, Englehardt's emphasis on the primacy of autonomy and his acceptance of the consequences of this emphasis are nothing new. In earlier work Englehardt follows the logic of his argument to its inevitable conclusions: "One must be willing, as a price for recognizing the freedom of others, to live with the consequences of that freedom: some persons will make choices that they would regret were they to live longer."[24]

When autonomy becomes the first condition of morality, one must be willing to tolerate exercises of autonomy with which one may personally disagree and feel impelled by conscience to oppose. Hence, in his book Englehardt must argue for the rightness of the consequences of his system—infanticide, abortion, assisting suicide, and direct euthanasia.

Despite the objections to this dangerous line of argument, one must grant the persuasive appeal of Englehardt's thesis. To object is to appear to discount the importance of human freedom. Yet in the end, from both a philosophical and a clinical point of view, the autonomy thesis as Englehardt rigorously proposes it fails.

First, the condition of possibility of morality is not freedom per se, but the freedom to articulate, defend, and pursue the good. This is certainly true for Kant, and for other moral thinkers as well. Freedom does not stand naked. It is clothed by an "ought"; we are free to do what we ought to do. A good case can be made that this is the original meaning of rights as well: a freedom to do what one is obliged to do, not an entitlement to specific treatment by others. While we agree that freedom is an important component in a pluralistic society, it should not be seen as the condition of morality. Rather, it is a component value among others. Thus, the greatest value of Englehardt's reasoning is that it constitutes the strongest argument against his premises. The logical consequences of autonomy as an absolute principle are as he says they are, but the unacceptability of his conclusions alerts the reader to the error of accepting the proposed first principle. Logic may lead us to the edge of the cliff, but before we step off, we should reexamine the starting point that led to this perilous state.[25]

Further, Englehardt repeatedly emphasizes the importance, indeed, the essentiality, of a peaceable society. He does not offer any reason to accept this laudable goal other than that such a society fosters autonomy and freedom. In his view these are the irreducible maxims of a decent human society. Yet this approach creates a circular argument. Autonomy is necessary for a peaceable society because a peaceable society is necessary for autonomy.

We believe Englehardt has erred. Most persons would observe that the real hallmark of a peaceable society is that it strikes a balance between fostering individual autonomy and limiting that autonomy for the common good. If everyone were free to ride roughshod over the values of others, society would collapse instantly. It would be the antithesis of peaceable. This is an important point, for it also bears on a better, more idealistic conception of autonomy.

There is another, less conventional way of looking at autonomy. In this view the self-regulation of autonomy is less important than its value for the humanity of persons. Autonomy is owed to humans as humans since it is a necessary condition for the operation of their humanity. Yet we live in a community in which we owe a limited autonomy to each other—not because of the absoluteness of our freedom, but because a decent human society is impossible if it violates the fundamental humanity of its citizens. In this view, similar to Aristotle's, ethics is a branch of politics, and autonomy is a gift given to one another for the sake of the common good.

Autonomy imposes at least two obligations: First, autonomy obliges us to use our freedom wisely in determining what we ought to do (often called an individual's conscience). Second, autonomy obliges us to use our freedom to advance the good society, a society that maximizes the good and welfare of all its citizens. Accordingly, autonomy cannot be used for ends that are inimical to intrinsic goods of individuals and society (to be discussed in later chapters) without moral peril. Absolute freedom, as Niebuhr pointed out, leads to the domination of the weak by the strong, the poor by the rich. One should foster a peaceable community not just to preserve freedom but also to develop the potentialities for a common, social existence as well.

With respect to medical ethics, other objections to Englehardt's autonomy thesis may be raised. Moral views arise from specific communities that develop definitions of the good based on their history and tradition. With this firm grounding, what ought to be done is defined and critiqued. The moral purpose of medicine is to serve the good of the patient. Englehardt's thesis is dangerously out of touch with this tradition in medicine.

Of course, what has been the case in the past is not necessarily valid for the present. Yet any critical reflection on beneficence must include limitations on autonomy. There are too many clinical situations in which freedom—either the physician's or the patient's—must be curtailed. In the real world of clinical medicine, there are no absolute moral principles except the injunction to act in the patient's best interests. Thus Veatch, who strongly supports the primacy of autonomy over beneficence in the relationship between doctor and patient, reluctantly admits the limits of autonomy in its ability to meet and address social needs. He therefore acknowledges that it is a "rare case" in which an "isolated patient [would] exercise his or her will unbounded by obligations to others."[26] In fact, besides social constraints on autonomy, there are also biological ones.[27] The possibilities for choice are only those "displayed before our consciousness."[28] In addition, illness itself impedes choices and actions.[29]

LIMITS OF AUTONOMY

Let us turn to some examples of the limits of autonomy that follow from our theory of relational good proposed in this chapter. We will examine further the principle of preservation of bodily good from these points of view: (1) What are licit decisions for the patient? (2) What are licit decisions for the physician? And (3) How should conflicts between physician and patient be resolved?

Autonomy would be wrongly exercised if it rejected penicillin treatment for pneumococcal or meningococcal meningitis. Both infections are life threatening and possess a high potential for central nervous system damage if the patient does recover. The same would be true of rejecting surgery for a ruptured spleen, appendicitis, or a subdural hematoma. Here the capabilities of medicine are both effective and beneficial.

At the other end of the spectrum, we can think of marginal treatments—those offering temporary, slight, or questionable benefit—that might, in varying degrees, be burdensome and expensive. The same treatments mentioned above, if considered for a dying patient, might represent a disproportion between burden and benefit.[30] Under these conditions one could choose to reject the good of the body in favor of other goods—saving one's own or one's family's money, or forestalling pain, discomfort, loss of dignity, and so on.

The difficulties would lie between these extremes. Definitions of effectiveness and benefit in relation to bodily good will, of course, be a matter for negotiation between the doctor and the patient, as mentioned in the previous chapter. But, as in all middle situations, one might fall on one or the other side depending on how the benefits-to-burdens calculus is determined. The benefits are sometimes hard to delineate with certainty, while the burdens are often too clear.

From the patient's point of view, then, it would be morally licit to reject useless or marginal treatments, or even those that are effective but not beneficial, that is, in the patient's best interests. One can, for example, effectively treat bacterial pneumonia in a patient dying inexorably from metastatic malignant disease. But such treatment would not be beneficial to the person, or even to the biological good of his or her body, since it only prolongs dying or suffering. On the other hand, one could conceive of a good transcending biological good, for example a patient wanting life prolonged so his family can be with him in his last moments. In this circumstance treating the patient's pneumonia is both effective and beneficial.

When treatments are, without reservations, biologically good and beneficial, we would favor treatment as a moral obligation for both the patient and the physician. We may favor other goods when treatment is only marginally effective or beneficial. Essentially, our position is that preserving the health of the body is a good, and we have a moral obligation to sustain it except under special circumstances in which biological good may be superseded.

But what about the doctor? To what extent can he or she cooperate with the patient's autonomous decision when by so doing the patient acts in a way that frustrates the good of the body, that is, when effective and beneficial treatment is rejected? For the patient, as we will argue later in this book, there is a hierarchy of values in which medical good, the good of the body, can be the lowest good. Thus, from the patient's point of view, a Jehovah's Witness can reject a blood transfusion because of a higher good—the patient's spiritual destiny as he or she sees it. On purely naturalistic grounds this patient is acting morally. If the doctor disagrees and forces the patient to be transfused, he violates the patient's humanity—a good higher than the good of the body. Here we disagree with Ramsey's medical indications policy, which would seem to require that the patient accept the treatment just because it is medially indicated.

In the first instance the doctor might agree that he could "cooperate" with the patient, especially if he accords a higher value to the spiritual realm than to bodily health. On the other hand, the doctor might disagree if he sees no validity in spiritual values and, indeed, rejects them as romantic nonsense. Alternatively, the doctor might place the highest weight on spiritual values and, on this ground, reject the patient's choice against transfusion because the physician feels there is a spiritual duty to preserve life and the health of the body until it is God's will that they be terminated—the Orthodox Jewish position. In this latter instance the physician cannot cooperate with what, in terms of his own spiritual belief system, is evil.

Depending upon how strongly the doctor holds this belief and how serious he deems the harm to the patient, he must make a decision: to withdraw from the case, deciding that such an act is evil but does not require intervention; to stay with the patient, passively not doing what he believes ought to be done because he deems protecting the patient's autonomy a higher good; or to stay with the patient because he deems the action such that it would be immoral to withdraw from the case. Rather, the doctor might decide that to preserve his own moral integrity he must intervene by, for example, treating the patient against his will if possible, deceiving the patient into thinking he will not treat him, or intervening by obtaining a court order overriding the patient's wishes. (The unlikelihood today of such a court order regarding a competent patient does not remove the moral dilemma for the doctor.)

What are the moral obligations of doctors and all others who witness what they think is seriously immoral? What are the ethical conditions for morally defensible interventions? Are there any? Does a morally defensible procedure for decision making override the substance of the decision? Are there some decisions that autonomous patients are not free to make in a democratic pluralistic society? Is Engelhardt right in claiming that the interest of maintaining a peaceable society takes precedence over even the most strongly held religious beliefs? It is true that, given the choice, the restraint must be upon individuals who would restrain those who they consider wrongdoers? Have we lost a common consensus on morals to such a degree that there is no longer any community of values? Are there any values in common other than autonomy? What are they? One look at the abortion debate quickly disabuses us of any hope of reconciliation. Granting that bombing abortion clinics is wrong because it perpetrates serious harm to do good, what measures are morally licit if one seriously believes that abortion clinics are the sites of mass murder? Are they any different from Auschwitz? We did take arms against Auschwitz, and did ourselves bomb, maim, and burn to eradicate its evil. We did harm to bring about good.

We are not arguing for bombing abortion clinics, but how far can private morality be allowed to go before it erodes the cement that holds human society together? Are there any things that ought never be done privately in a good society? Can a society survive such radical pluralism that there are no longer any shared values?

The answer to these difficult questions seem to lie in the system C approach we delineated at the start of this chapter. Consider autonomy and paternalism two forms of the same sort of an ethics of individualism. In this ethic the self is primary and the root of all ethical decision making. Value is placed on the self-consciousness of all beings. To be retarded, a fetus, or an incompetent Alzheimer's patient is to be disvalued in this system. Justifications must be developed to transfer the respect for persons given to self-conscious entities to these unfortunate beings. Self-determination and liberty are the primary values. Society is seen in a libertarian way as a mechanism for protecting, as far as possible, individual liberties, even if these appear wrongheaded or downright offensive and evil to others. This is certainly the view proposed by Englehardt. We perceive no real difference between the autonomy and medical paternalism models in these respects. Both models emphasize individual decision making; both emphasize the freedom from constraint that society might place on individuals. For the autonomy model the freedom is that of the patient; for the paternalism model, that of the physician.

Contrast this individualistic view with a community-based ethics. In the latter the emphasis and highest values are placed on the person in relation to others. The fetus is seen as partly related to its mother and father; the retarded is seen as a community member, regardless of intellectual function; the Alzheimer's patient a true person, not a former person lacking the mark of self-consciousness needed to be a person. In this view, not autonomy but beneficence predominates. The important thing for persons to do for one another is to act compassionately, anticipate and meet each other's needs, and form the important bonds among them that may transcend rational analysis. Care for others is reinforced by society; rather than simply protecting individuals from encroachments on their freedom, individuals are encouraged and positively reinforced in their interventions to help others.

Of course, both sketches are slighted for reasons of space. We do not wish to imply that individualists, as we have described them, would necessarily fight for the rights of child pornographers who link such pornography with the joys of the serial murder of children (after all, there are some limits on individual freedoms). Similarly, we would not want to imply that all communalists, if we may call them that, would intervene "helpfully" in the lives of others to such an extent that they would become obnoxious, as reportedly were the Calvinistic founders of the Massachusetts colony. Nevertheless, the metaethical approach one takes on either of these two models predetermines the choices to be made in specific instances.

We have argued that medicine as a human activity lies between these two extremes. Its focus in the clinical setting is on the individual. Yet there are limits, set by the body's needs and society's expectations, on the autonomous decisions to be made by both patient and physician. Further, the relation between doctor and patient establishes a community of dialogue. As Marzuk suggests, excessive concern for patient autonomy, the hectic pace of modern medicine, and the litigious environment of society itself lead physicians to become, at worst, cautious about persuading patients to do what is in their best interests and, at best, noncommittal.[31] These fears and pressures, naturally enough, stifle the important dialogue about values that is the centerpiece of a beneficent model of medicine. Recall that such negotiation is required because no one value predominates in advance, though the principle of acting in the best interest of the patient guides the discussion. Being cautious and noncommittal about what is best for the patient forecloses this essential negotiating process.

Finally the "communal event" is based on the biological and social needs of the patient as well. We have suggested, in order to avoid the universality of the World Health Organization definition of health, that the primary method by which physicians help construct healing is through the body. Since that body is both biological ("It hurts in my chest") and social ("I am under stress"), the physician is involved with fundamental human values. These values bridge individualistic and community-based ethical systems.

A theory of the good in medicine provides an ordering principle whereby conflicts between social and individual good, between autonomy and beneficence, can be resolved. Such a theory is requisite also for ordering the physician's obligations, which are necessary both to the individual and to society. When these are in conflict—as they increasingly can be when resources are scarce and personal and communal definitions of the good society confront each other—the physician needs to place his or her obligations in some priority relationship. We will examine that system of priorities in the chapters to come. In the next chapter, however, we develop our beneficence theory against the backdrop of the fiduciary relationship between doctor and patient.

4

Beneficence-in-Trust

Almost everyone who has pondered the dialectical opposition of autonomy and paternalism has seen that a new model of the doctor-patient relationship is needed. Two models now compete for dominance in such a resolution: The first stresses the contractual nature of the relation; the second, only now emerging, stresses the fiduciary nature of the physician-patient interaction.

In this chapter we will first sketch the background for the contractual model and the initial development of the fiduciary model, and then will present our model of beneficence-in-trust as a further development of the fiduciary model.

CONTRACTUAL AND FIDUCIARY MODELS

The contractual model of the doctor-patient relationship was born in response to traditional paternalism and in support of the autonomy theory of decision making in health care. Traditionally, medical ethics has been grounded in the relation of doctor and patient. This provides both an anchor for the philosophical discussion within the clinical domain of medicine and, simultaneously, a starting point for the development of philosophy of medicine itself.[1]

Proposals for the contractual model have gone through changes over the past ten years. At first they were based almost totally on the patient's right to make decisions. While this emphasis was probably needed to counteract the vigor of traditional medical paternalism, the model was seriously flawed. As Veatch notes in his own "celebration" of the death of the Hippocratic ethic, "For one thing it [the patient rights model] focused almost exclusively on the rights of patients, saying nothing about the rights of health care professionals. For another it did little to overcome the individualism of the earlier Hippocratic ethic."[2] In other words, the earlier contractual models were developed to fight against the relative power differential between physician and patient left over from an overly paternalistic interpretation of the relationship.

But by the time Fried addressed the question, he tried to accommodate two elements from the tradition as well as two elements from a rights ethic. He called these the "rights of personal care." Lucidity and autonomy, full disclosure and self-determination, respectively, were the features borrowed from the rights ethic. Retained from the earlier tradition, however, were fidelity and humanity. Fried defined fidelity as the right to continuing service aimed at one's own interests, and the rejection of possibly conflicting interests. He defined humanity as the right to be treated with compassion.[3] The latter two features are obviously derived from beneficence, while the former seem to follow from autonomy.

Similarly, Veatch's struggle over the years to find a suitable model for the relation led him to reject three others, leaving him only with the contractual model. He rejects the priestly model because of its liberal dose of paternalism. Also rejected are the engineering model and the collegial model; the former assumes that patients can direct the physician even regarding technical matters, and the latter assumes that both parties are equal in technical matters. Neither is the case. The contractual model, then, was presented as a compromise. In it the physician would retain goals and values regarding technical matters, while the patient would retain power over all matters of personal values.[4]

Veatch's later work spelled out how the contractual model rested not just on negotiation between the doctor and the patient but on Rawls' theory of a social contract.[5] He argues, as we do, that what is needed is an ethic "that avoids paternalism"; he is further concerned, though, with avoiding individualism and consequentialism. As he says, "Specifying these principles would require participation by both professionals and lay people and eventually spell out the duties as well as the rights of both groups."[6]

In general, contractual models are criticized for several reasons. First, even though Veatch recognizes that both physician and patient have interests, he tends to limit the physician's interests to technical matters. In this, in our view, he too severely limits the humanity of the physician. Second, the supposed "death" of the Hippocratic ethic is really no more than an overcoming of the paternalistic interpretation of that ethic. Granting that excesses have occurred, a more balanced historical account of the tradition would center on two features to be retained in current models: the act of profession by the physician and the fact of illness in the patient.[7] Third, the contractual model seems to rest on an inaccurate assumption. Physicians and patients, in fact, rarely discuss their contract in the explicit terms required by Veatch's approach.[8] A fourth criticism can be leveled against a rights ethic itself. Thinking of the doctor-patient relation as a contract seems to establish only minimal expectations from the physician and the patient. The physician will deal with the technical values; the patient will deal with personal and social values. In reality things are much more complex than this.

A number of thinkers have begun to develop a richer model, one that can be called the *fiduciary model*. This is certainly the case for the negotiation described by Katz in *The Silent World of the Doctor and Patient*.[9] In order to overcome that silence, a mutual dialogue about values and techniques must take place. The model presented by Katz does not artificially delimit either the physician's humanity or the patient's quest to understand possible medical interventions.

A second source for a richer model can be one in which a sort of fiduciary paternalism is developed. In this model, professionals are to intervene in a patient's life in order to bring about greater eventual autonomy. Moody has developed this model as an alternative to utilitarian or consequentialist concerns. Rather than protecting patients from themselves, professionals would develop strategies for reinforcing autonomous choice in patients and, if need be, would protect them in carrying out such choices.[10] Moody contrasts this sort of paternalism, as he calls it, with a best-interests paternalism, in which the health professional decides what is best for the patient. What is important for this discussion is Moody's recognition that Childress' approach to paternalism and autonomy is based on rules, guidelines, procedures, and strictures. He, like Katz, bases his own proposal on "virtues exhibited by the professional in conditions of ambiguity or conflict: on capacities for wisdom, insight, discretion, self-criticism, and so on."[11]

A fiduciary model such as the one we will propose is based on a rediscovery of the ethic of virtue rather than an ethic of rules. A number of insights lead to this rediscovery. The first is that an ethic of rules alone cannot provide guarantees that the responsible individual, the person with duties, will carry out those rules. That person must have the kind of character that disposes him to act in accordance with the right rules of actions.[12,13] He must be the kind of person who can be trusted.

Second, as MacIntyre argues so cogently, the effort to establish ethics on a post-Enlightenment system of rules and principles is fatally flawed. There can be no "bottom line" thinking in ethics.[14] The objection that the ethics of virtue reduces ethics solely to the habits or dispositions of individuals can be met by providing guidelines for actions—certain axioms that derive, in turn, from communities of practice. One such community is the relationship established by patients and physicians.

Any approach grounded in trust should include the possibility of negotiation as the relationship continues and progresses. Such negotiation enables both physician and patient to continuously reexamine their values. Siegler makes this point a major component in his effort to detail what we conceive to be the moral certainty of medicine. He notes that "if moral certainty exists in medicine (that is, if it is possible to determine which actions taken in a medical context are moral and ethical, which are right and wrong), such moral certainty will be discovered not by recourse to formal laws, moral rules, or moral principles, but rather in the context of the particularities of the physician-patient relationship itself."[15]

In addition, a fiduciary model should rest on treating the whole person. The reason is that the values of the patient must also be part of the dialogue about medical treatment. No less a thinker than Plato saw the importance of this "current" need: "This is the great error of our day that physicians separate the soul from the body. The cure of the part should not be attempted without the treatment of the whole, and also that no attempt should be made to cure the body without the soul."[16]

Finally, such a model should incorporate what we have termed the *moral center* of medicine. Originally, this conception had to do with the paradigm case that could clearly circumscribe the heart and soul of medical practice. But is has now come to mean the interaction itself, with all of the human joys and sorrows. It is not merely a contract. It is not merely a philosophical entity. It is not merely a transaction between autonomous parties. Jonsen and Jameton describe the elements of the moral center as an effort to heal within the context of a petitioner coming with a complaint and a professional who promises to heal.[17] This is also our thesis.

Such a relationship is established through deliberate acts by both physicians and patients. It has within it what we have called a particular vulnerability of the patient, which the professional must address.[18] The ideal of working on behalf of the patient, then, as Fried notes, "implies an interest and a right on the part of the doctor as well to maintain the integrity of his activity, to work not as a tool or as the bureaucratic agent of a social system, but as one whose professional activity is a personal expression of his own nature."[19] With regard to these and other features, recall the axioms of the beneficence model we formulated at the end of chapter 3.

Finally, this approach should be based on a theory of the patient's good. In the next chapter we will spell out this good, arguing, as did Kass, that the health functioning of the organism as a whole "is not just the absence of disease, but a positive good and the proper norm for medical practice."[20]

BENEFICENCE-IN-TRUST

In chapter 5, we argued that no one principle of ethics could govern all health care practice. Yet we also proposed that beneficence should be the fundamental principle guiding medical care. We further noted that the principle of beneficence joined concern for the best interests of patients with concern for their autonomy. As a result the principle takes on the character of a shorthand that conflates two very important ethical concerns in medicine, autonomy and beneficence. Only in this way can it function as a "single" principle. We have stressed the differences between this conception of beneficence and the usual characterizations of autonomy of the patient and the utilitarian nature of paternalism. By extracting beneficence from the mix of concerns that swirl around the practice of medicine, we have developed an inductive methodology within a philosophy of medicine.

We call this sort of beneficence, one that encompasses several other ethical principles, *beneficence-in-trust*. By beneficence-in-trust we mean that physicians and patients hold "in trust" (Latin, *fiducia*) the goal of acting in the best interests of one another in the relationship. In the main, the patient's fulfillment of this trust resides in carrying out the negotiated plan for his or her health. The burden of trust more often belongs on the physician, who must act in the best interests of the patient under the conditions we have already discussed, including social conditions.

Negotiation, then, does indeed occur in the doctor-patient relationship. But this negotiation is guided by beneficence. Negotiation is important, but it does not establish patient good per se, or the end of medicine—the fact of illness and act of profession. Siegler's notion seems to base the negotiaton on dialogue alone rather than on the nature of the relationship itself. The latter establishes an onto-logical bond of need and response. Both doctor and patient, in order to fulfill the objectives of the relation, must act in the best interests of the patient. Extramedical values may intrude on this relationship, and sometimes may over-ride beneficence for other temporarily important matters, as we shall see.

In everyday circumstances, for example, the primary duty of the physician is to the patient. However, if a crisis occurs in the allocation of medical care due to a bomb blast, an explosion, a fire, an earthquake, or other catastrophe, the physician is obligated to act in the best interests of preserving the community. Hence, when the bomb fell in Hiroshima, the first duty of all the citizens was to save those who could help restore order and return life to "normal." Note that the social triage principle does not target for salvage only those persons who obtained social merit during or before the catastrophe, but rather those who can best get things running again afterwards. Only in such extreme cases is the phy-sician justified in abandoning the principle of beneficence in favor of another principle.

But overriding beneficence does not occur when physicians respect the wishes of patients. In this regard the American Board of Internal Medicine describes the ideal characteristics of the internist as compassion, integrity, and respect for the wishes of patients.[21] Respecting wishes of patients is an essential feature of acting in their best interests. These qualities closely parallel ancient descriptions of physicians as possessed of *compassio, professio, and humanitas.*[22]

Nor does acting in the best interests of patients override autonomy or con-stitute paternalism. Beneficence, as we have described it, cannot contribute to paternalism (as Childress once seemed to think) because it cannot be based on a violation of so fundamental an element of humanity as patient preferences. Take as an example the New Jersey Supreme Court "tests" that were offered for making judgments about incompetent patients. The court, in the *Conroy* case, proposed the following tests.

The Subjective Test

In this test, one attempts to obtain the presumed wishes of the patient from a guardian and then follows them. The patient does not lose the right to refuse or request treatment just because he or she loses competence. Hence, respecting the presumed wishes of the patient is a form of honoring her autonomy, even though she may suffer from an irreversible condition that renders her incompetent. The court makes it clear that one cannot employ a standard by which one treats patients according to what other persons might think is reasonable (the reasonable person criterion) but, rather, according to ascertainable preferences of the patient.

When one cannot with some certainty discover the wishes of the incompetent patient, one may turn to the benefits-to-burdens calculus. At first blush this appears to be a form of utilitarianism. But this is not the case since the emphasis is on a patient's own preferences and, in their absence, on acting in the best interest of the patient.

The Limited Objective Test

In the absence of reliable, "trustworthy" information about possible preferences of the patient, one may act on probable wishes in conjunction with a judgment that the burdens of the treatment outweigh the benefit of continued life to the patient.

The Pure Objective Test

In the absence of any information about a patient's preferences, one may discontinue treatment on two grounds, both of which must be present. First, the benefits-to-burdens calculus, as described in the limited objective test, may be used, but, second, only if the burden of treatment can be considered cruel or inhumane.[23] Put another way, in the absence of a patient's expression of wishes, or advance directives, or a guardian's reliable report of wishes, one must act on the basis of medical indications (or medical good) unless these prove cruel, painful, and unless given the nature of the patient's medical problems.

In our view the New Jersey Supreme Court applied a model of beneficence-in-trust. Held in trust in the relationship with an incompetent patient are two duties of beneficence: one to honor previous wishes, and the other not to harm the patient by disproportionate care, that is, burdensome care that is futile. The former duty is based on respect for autonomy. The latter is based on the best interests of the patient, not as we might view his or her life from our vantage point, but as it must proceed in its current state.

In this model we do not so much judge the quality of life ("this kind of life cannot be worth living") as the "hopeless" relation between burdens and benefits. In balancing burdens and benefits, one must make some determination about the status of a given person's life at the time the judgment or comparison between burdens and benefits is made.

But this determination does not aim at the worth of a person's life. Rather, it clarifies the status of his or her existence at this time. It tries to ascertain, as prudently as possible, what action will most benefit the patient. The question is not so much whether or not she is a person (and what duties we might have toward beings who once were persons but are no longer), but what medically justifiable actions we propose to take given the patient's current and forseeable condition. Using beneficence in trust, the physician does not calculate the relation of the person's life to society's judgment of the value of that person, but instead calculates the relation of medical treatments to the patient's condition and prognosis.[24] Some treatments would thus be considered out of porportion to the benefits that might accrue to the patient. Ultimately, one calculates the impact of the proposed intervention on the fiduciary commitment of the doctor to serve the best interests of his or her patient within the structures imposed by the patient's clinical state.

Paternalism is often justified by appeal to maximizing the welfare of all, while the doctrine of autonomy is justified by appeal to respect for persons. These two principles inevitably clash in medical practice. Beauchamp and McCullough discerned the same conflict, but contrasted beneficence and autonomy rather than paternalism and autonomy:

> The conflict generated by the two models [that is, beneficence and autonomy] is an inescapable dimension of medical practice: a conflict between the patient's best interests understood from the perspective of medicine and the patient's best interests understood from the perspective of the patient. . . . The upshot is that the obligations generated by these models are all *prima facie,* . . . all moral principles seem noble and inviolable when stated free of conflict with other principles. But controversial problems for medical ethics arise when their applicability in circumstances of conflict must be determined. A central task of medical ethics is thus to fix the limits of each of the two models in light of the demands of the other.[25]

We agree that there is a conflict, but the conflict is between paternalism and autonomy, not beneficence and autonomy. As we have argued, beneficence can function as the resolution point for conflicts that do arise between the doctor's and the patient's view of the good for the patient is always the medical good, that is, the medically indicated course of action. This is too circumscribed a notion of the physician's role in the doctor-patient relation, and too narrow a view of the patient's good. The physician must also contemplate and negotiate other values in the patient's hierarchy of goods.

We suggest, rather, that there is a third principle in medicine that we have called beneficence-in-trust. It secures the autonomy of patients, unlike paternalism, which regards patient autonomy as inimical to best interests, especially when the patient does not agree with the physician. In this way, fiduciary beneficence underlies the role of the physician as an advocate for the patient, or even as his proxy or surrogate in cases of incompetence when no prior wishes are known and no other proxies are available.

With respect to the more difficult conflict between beneficence and social welfare, our proposal is less a resolution of the conflict than a frank admission of its existence, with some ideas for minimizing that conflict. Individual and social good will almost always clash in a cost-cutting environment. Morreim

calls this "learning to live with the inevitable," suggesting that the mutual expectations of the physician and patient must be revised. In her view the physician
can no longer expect to provide "everything" for the patient; neither can the
patient expect to obtain "everything" from the physician. She argues that "the
physician need not promise to do "everything" in order to promise to do his
very best. He need not pretend that his own patients' needs preempt the needs
of other patients and the requirements of justice, in order to give his own
patients a position of very special priority with their relationship."[26] We are not
convinced that the patient's needs should not be primary, but this point deserves
the sort of amplification we provide later.

We have suggested that persons should be required to plan their health care
in advance. During discussion with their physicians, they can receive more guidance on how to ensure that their decision-making autonomy can be preserved.
If patients do find, before treatment begins, that it is difficult to articulate their
wishes, physician's then have the opportunity to educate them about the scope
of treatments and their impact on the body and on prolonging life. The more
these decisions can be made in advance, the greater the change that beneficence
will not be violated in the relationship, and that sufficient resources will remain
so that other citizens may have an equal opportunity to make decisions about
their health.

As O'Rourke observes in his newest work on medical ethics, "Medicine
works only where there is a cooperative and consensual relationship between
patients and professionals."[27] Most ethicists and physicians would agree with his
and our own endorsement of the need for negotiation. Thus, Smith and Churchill, writing about primary care, stress that they

> wish to affirm the person-centered character of medical ethics; that princi-
> ples and rules reflect our assumptions about what relationships (and the
> people who form them) should be like. Hence, to jump from problems to
> principles or rules, and then to solutions, does violence to the very stuff that
> makes moral problems what they are. Medical-ethical problem-solving is
> not a generalizable and repeatable exercise in logic; it is an examination of
> the moral motivations and sensibilities which constitute us as "doctor" or
> "patient."[28]

In a very different but equally important vein, Hauerwas underscores the
importance of the doctor-patient relationship, not as a contract between autonomous entities (in which the temptation to construe medical care as property
becomes almost irresistible), but as a dialogue of caring and a vehicle for
"uncovering some of our most profound moral commitments as a
community."[29]

II

THE IMPLICATIONS OF BENEFICENCE FOR THE DOCTOR AND PATIENT

5

Health and Ethical Norms

We have argued that a theory of beneficence can surmount the difficulties inherent in the patient autonomy or medical paternalism models for the doctor-patient relation. Further, we have suggested that beneficence is well suited to medicine because it expresses the values inherent in medical theory and practice better than ethical theories based in either rights or social benefits. Still further, we have pointed out that beneficence is the guiding moral principle in the relation between physician and patient, that is, acting for the best interests of the patient.

At this stage of our argument, the next task is to define how health can be a value and, as such, function as the basis of norms in the doctor-patient relation. It is erroneous, in our view, to claim that all aspects of clinical decisions are negotiable or relative. Some goods are more important than others and cannot be violated without destroying the purpose of medicine itself. One of these is healing. Nonetheless, some goods we will identify in the next chapter entirely transcend the medical relationship and are often much more significant for the patient and health profession than medical ones. What is nonnegotiable is what is normative in the relation between doctor and patient. Our argument will clarify the way in which health can be both a nonnegotiable and a negotiable value in the doctor-patient relationship.

Goods or values enter medicine in several ways: (1) in the concepts of health and disease; (2) insofar as medicine is the art of healing; (3) insofar as medicine is itself a habit of making decisions that are good for the patient, and (4) finally, since a concept of good underlies every professional act, these goods or values interact with each other and with other goods or values extrinsic to medicine. These various values must be brought into some balanced relationship with each other at the moment of actual decision making.

To establish such a relationship, we must ask the central question, does the commitment to healing impose different standards of morality on health professionals as compared with others in society? Are there role-specific duties? In this chapter we will argue that being a health professional does make a moral difference.

HEALTH AS A VALUE

Though health can be interpreted in a variety of ways, one interpretation is as the biological good of a living organism: that is, health is efficient biological functioning. The idea "It is good to be healthy" functions as a norm in medical decisions. It is in this connection that we have stated, "As a fundamental need of living organisms, health can be said to be an absolute intrinsic value."[1] The normative status of health can be properly identified as a "biological need of living organisms." We agree with Sadegh-zadeh that health may become a relative value in the actual decisions patients make.[2] That is a point we shall develop in the next chapter. Patients may value other goods over health—pleasure, travel, wealth, prestige, independence from physicians, or family togetherness. They may then reject the doctor's recommendations even when he or she aims at a broad or "holistic" conception of health. The physician may wish to incorporate other individual and social values in his goal of treatment. But the patient may negate these also by refusing the medically indicated treatment.

Clinical decisions derive their special quality from the interrelationship of three phenomena: the fact of illness, the act of medicine, and the act of profession.[3] Health is what the patient expects; health is what the physician professes to restore; health is the aim of the healing decision and the act of medicine; the loss of health characterizes the fact of illness. The norm "It is good to be healthy" governs the three interacting phenomenological desiderata of an authentic medical transaction.

Health, therefore, functions prescriptively in a medical decision insofar as it is the good toward which both patient and physician aspire. Indeed, without health as its end, the medical relationship would never be initiated. Nor would it be a medical relationship since decisions about goods other than health can be, and are, better made outside the physician-patient relationship.

We do not claim, therefore, that health is always, and in all human decisions, an absolute prescriptive value or that it would always take precedence over other values. To repeat, health is for us a prescriptive value in the medical transaction as we have defined it, and within that carefully drawn phenomenological context it is a primary value.

To make the claim that health is a primary value within the doctor-patient relation immediately creates two problems. First, does health have any value in the realm of those forms of preventive medicine in which no specific doctor-patient relation exists? Obviously, it does. In preventive medicine, when a direct threat exists to the health of the population, health functions as a social good imposed on (and therefore not necessarily valued by) individuals. A good example is the effort by public health officials to induce homosexuals with AIDS to refrain from sexual activities in order to protect others. In other cases, in which the threat is less clearly established or when no teeth exist in laws to enforce the good, health is an optional social good. In cases like these, health was formerly seen as more of a social than an individual value in preventive medicine. It was assigned to a different place in a calculus of goods than in a one-to-one doctor-patient relation.[4] This is less true at present since more and more individuals take charge of their own fitness and health.

The second problem created by claiming that health is a primary value in the doctor-patient relation has more to do with the thesis of this book. A patient's or doctor's value rankings may vary with changes in any of the following: life situation, the range of available alternatives, the criteria for making assessments, perception, and ultimate moral principles. These variables interact in the ranking of values in medical decisions. They are critically important for understanding the place of health in a hierarchy of values. In relation to the factors we mentioned and many others, health can be a relative, extrinsic value because it is a means to an end as well as an end, or it can shift its place in the relative ranking of values. In any case, we hold that health is "primary" in the doctor-patient relationship insofar as a definite stand must be taken on its importance to the patient within that relation.

In order to clarify the ways in which health may function as a value, we propose a brief axiology for medicine. Axiology is that branch of philosophy that deals formally and systematically with values, and such a mapping of values has been, for the most part, implicit in medical writings and practice. An axiologic analysis should make the role of values in medicine much more explicit.

In what specific ways can the proposition "health is a value" be understood? We will show that, at a minimum, health may be considered as individual or social, intrinsic or extrinsic, absolute or preventive, and systemic or nonsystemic.

Health as a Social Value

It is clear that health has a *social* value since society sanctions the use of public funds to support health care programs such as sanitation, vaccination, and health care insurance. In these instances health is considered an ideal and an objective of a good society. It is difficult to conceive of a healthy society whose citizens are not also healthy. Health is a value since it is a community aim with respect to an obtainable good. There is a moral mandate to work for this good since it is obtainable for at least a certain amount of time and for most citizens. Thus, the first way in which health can be taken as a value is as an obtainable good for the community.

In this context health is a *relative* good with respect to other fundamental needs of human life, but an *absolute* good for those programs designed to achieve the specific aim of public health or social medicine. The "act of profession" in this case is a promise by the public health agency to achieve the objective of community health. As a promise, it cannot be subverted without inflicting an injustice on the whole community. Health is thus a moral good. It is, therefore, a moral as well as a social value. Judged within the framework of public health, health carries an *absolute* normative function. If it is ignored by those who profess to be public health providers, the failure is moral as well as political.

Health is a relative value when a society ranks it among other social values—security, jobs, national defense, housing, and the like. Here society is choosing among aims and objectives, and health may be more or less valued in different times and places. Once it is chosen as a social aim, it becomes an *absolute* normative value for those who profess to fulfill that aim for society. Health can be either a relative or an absolute value, depending upon the decision-making context.

Health as an Individual Value

Health can be taken as a value for the individual in three ways. The first encompasses health as an *absolute* value of the living body through which a person exists. The person may or may not value health consciously, but the body "protoselects" health.[5] The smoker and drinker who quit find that, within limits, the lungs and liver will repair the damage over a period of years. The body left to itself tends to heal; this is the ancient *vis medicatrix naturae.* The body is a self-regulating, self-restoring system that undergoes gradual functional impairment with age, but even then tends to restoration with whatever mechanisms are still intact. This is true even of the diseased organ or body that tends to repair injury or to maintain function.

Health is the end toward which the living body as a biological organism tends, and it is in this sense that it becomes an absolute intrinsic value of the living body. Health is a biological and ontological need for living bodies because without it the living body ultimately becomes something else—a corpse. In the end this need is frustrated by the eventual inevitable death of the organism. Disease is an ontological assault that the body works to reverse through its defense mechanisms. Philosophically speaking, then, health is not only a relative social good but an absolute good that must be sought in the act of profession of medicine when one person who lacks health seeks the assistance of another who promises to heal that defect.[6]

The second way health can be taken as a value for the individual is as a subjective or objective state of affairs. Health can be construed as a state of affairs within an agent's existence about which the agent may have preferences. it may be ranked above or below other values, and its moral weight may change with time, life experiences, perception, or convictions.

The subject counts himself or herself ill when some sign or symptom, sudden or gradual, is perceived to have effected a change in existential status—from feeling well to feeling ill. In the case of a stroke, an accident, or chest pain, the perception is immediate; in the case of a chronic symptom such as headache, subtle weight loss, or weakness, the perception may be so gradual that the transition in states cannot be definitively marked. In either case, however, it is the agent's perception of an existentially changed state of affairs that signals the lack of health. The absence of health then becomes a disvalue. At the moment at which help is contemplated or sought, the person becomes a patient; this is the first moment of clinical medicine, that moment when the patient herself feels the need for the helping or healing relationship.

It is at this point, too, that health can be viewed for the individual as an objective state of affairs. Someone else—a layman friend, a family member, or a professional—perceives objective changes in bodily or behavioral presence that signal a changed state of affairs. This might precede, be simultaneous with, or follow the patient's subjective perception. But, in any case, the judgment is one of experience, not of preference. Health here has a value as a *criterion*, as an objective measure of a changed state of affairs. The judgments of the observer are comparative with the subject's observed prior state of affairs or the state of affairs of all other human beings.

The third way health can be taken as a value for the individual occurs when a person enters the healing relationship, that is, when she perceives her illness to require the help of another person or persons, a professional or lay, regular or irregular practitioner. Here a very complex interaction occurs between a wide variety of sources of valuation for health—social, cultural, psychological, scientific, biological, and religious. Each source operates in each of the interacting subjects—patient, physician, nurse, and everyone who touches in any way on the patient's consciousness of her altered state of existence.

We note that all concepts of health and disease have value components. In the case of mental illness, what is disvalued in one culture may be valued in another. Engelhardt has shown how disease classifications are rooted in sociocultural determinants. As Engelhardt further points out, masturbation was considered a mental disease in the nineteenth century. It is possible to select symptoms and signs so that a disease may be included in or excluded from a classificatory schema.[7] Whether or not a disease will be in a classification will depend upon how one selects signs and symptoms to define the disease. The scientific and actuarial decisions that form the background of diagnosis are value laden as well, and are often shaped by the need to optimize outcomes for patients. These scientific decisions have variable moral weight, but they are never completely nonmoral since the end of the entire medical transaction is the good of the patient.

With these considerations in hand, we return to the point about mutual valuation of health and healing. The most important dimension of health as a value for individuals occurs in the healing relationship. Presumably, the patient seeks out a physician to assist in restoring health, and usually the definition of health is in large part the patient's. It is enhanced or modified by the physician's conception as well. Both physician and patient place a value or disvalue on choices of diagnostic, therapeutic, and healing procedures. How much pain, disability, and disturbance of life-style are tolerable to attain a certain health goal? What is the value of length versus quality of life? What is the goal of treatment: to cure, promote life, relieve pain, or gain time for some other purpose the patient identifies? The value questions are many. How they are answered turns on two things: what the doctor and patient think health *is*, and what value each places on its attainment. There may be conflicting interpretations about health as an individual value. The moral component is high because the physician or other professed healer promises to seek the *good* of the patient, that is, to do the right and good thing.

We have shown that, at a minimum, health can be conceived as a value in several different ways: (1) as a social good; (2) as an absolute intrinsic need; (3) as a state of affairs extrinsically valued; (4) as a criterion for comparative judgments or statements of fact; (5) as a scientific concept; and (6) as all of the preceding modulated by social, cultural, and historical valuations and disvaluations. We conclude, therefore, that health as a value cannot be limited to states of affairs in the body. The result would be a truncated axiology deficient in the rich possibilities that a broader view of health as a value would allow.

THE ETHICAL CHARACTER OF PROFESSIONS

If one is to argue that health and/or healing, as goods within the doctor-patient relation, have nonnegotiable or normative force within that relation, then it is necessary to establish that persons within the relationship are bound by specific ethical obligations not necessarily binding for the rest of the population or for the same persons outside of that relationship. Duties specific to associations such as the doctor-patient relationship give them an ethical character. Our argument is that physicians and, indeed, patients do have specific duties within the healing relationship. As a consequence, being a health professional does make an ethical difference. That being a patient also makes such a difference is considered in Chapters 6 and 10.

Of the four major ways in which medicine possesses an ethical character, the first is established through a public promise. Public profession* of a commitment to heal establishes a promise to work for the good of the patient with respect to matters of health. Such a public professional commitment to beneficence creates at least two responses in the social arena.

Public Promise

First, the profession and state certify through their accreditation, licensure, and professional associations that the physician is trained and competent to act in

---

*Etymologically, *profession* stems from the Latin *professio*, a public oath of fealty, or turning over one's obedience and loyalty to another.

the best interests of others. (In our last chapter we will spell out the specific commitments that ought to be part of a public declaration.) Certification alone, however, does *not* substitute for a commitment to care for health. That is why the public act of taking an oath, whether Hippocratic or a modernized version, is so important. The conferring of a degree upon a physician, nurse, or other health professional may signify competence through a course of training. It is the public taking of the oath that signifies entry into the profession. Just because the current status of the professional pledge and a medical code of professional conduct is in a state of flux is not sufficient reason to dispense with the ceremony of the oath. By his or her oath, the physician "takes office," as it were, an office of beneficence. But even if no such oath is publicly taken, the very act of entering practice and offering oneself as a physician is itself a promise of beneficence.

Second, as a direct consequence of the public promise to care for a patient's health, citizens expect physicians to act in their best interests. Thus, the public oath or the setting up of a practice establishes two obligations not required of those outside the profession of health care—the first is competence and the second is the use of that competence for the patient's benefit. This is the twofold covenant that physicians enter into with society and individual patients.

Mutual Valuation

The public promise or covenant, however, is not the only way in which the ethical character of the doctor-patient relation is established. It may also arise through mutual valuation. Since both patient and physician ordinarily value healing, this value "stamps" the relation with an ethical character (given that health is a good).[8] This is the case because health and/or healing is a moral value. That is to say, to be healthy is a good essential to being a fully fulfilled human individual and an effective human social entity. Note that we do not claim that perfect wholeness will ever be achieved, only that persons in search of healing are engaging in an ethical activity.

Role-Specific Duties

A third argument for the ethical character of the medical relationship rests on neither the public act of profession nor the mutual valuation of health, but on the duty of a physician qua physician. This is the deontological basis of professional ethics. Kant based his ethics on the duty of persons to *function* as persons, not on an analysis of acts, motives, ends, or rewards for good conduct. The duty of physicians, however, would not follow from the nature of a person but from the social role of a health professional. Ramsey calls these duties "canons of loyalty" to patients or to health.[9] These special duties may lead one to argue that physicians must always place the good of the patient over other goods. The subject of social versus individual goods, however, needs further elaboration in subsequent chapters.

Condition of Freedom

Finally, health may be considered to function axiomatically in medicine as a formal condition of freedom. If freedom is an essential feature of a moral agent, lack of health can impede ethical decision making. Certain universal characteristics of disease (dependency on others to be cured, ontological assault on personhood, objectivization of the body, dissolution of the self as a unified dynamic construct, and so forth)[10] are clues to similar universal attributes of being healthy (independence of action, autonomy, subjectivization of the body, a unified self-construct). The aim of physician and patient for promoting the positive attributes and removing the negatives ones, as far as possible, is an ethical one, not just a medical one, because this act fosters and confirms patients as moral entities.

We conclude that concern for the health of patients, for those who suffer a potential or real lack of health, creates the ethical character of the profession. This ethical character requires conduct on the part of both participants in the doctor-patient relation not required of others, or of the same agents when they are outside that relationship.

TWO OBJECTIONS TO MEDICINE'S ETHICAL CHARACTER

A notable objection to the entire line of reasoning we have presented comes from Goldman's argument in *The Moral Foundations of Professional Ethics*.[11] Goldman holds that being a health professional makes no ethical difference; the profession is not governed by a set of moral principles different from, or in conflict with, a common moral framework.

Physicians and other professionals often assume that their profession is "strongly role-differentiated," that the roles of the professional exempt one from common moral rules. Thus Goldman claims physicians often violate the rule of truth-telling in favor of a "higher" principle—beneficence or acting for the good of a patient (in our terms such a principle could only be paternalism). The problem is not so much that practitioners violate their own codes, but that they assume their codes take priority over the autonomous rights of individuals. Goldman argues that physicians have no such exemption from common morality.

This point leads to Goldman's proposal for a common morality in society. It is a form of modified utilitarianism in which he borrows the notion that "rights trump goods" from Dworkin, a renowned authority in the philosophy of law. According to Goldman, rights are interests "protective of the integrity of the individual person." Despite the merits of social goods such as health and healing, Goldman might assert, individual patient rights will always take priority over goods, even if those goods are the backbone of the profession of medicine. He is willing to admit that some rights are more important than others, and thus the political process must try to resolve clashes of rights. But he consistently argues that social goods cannot be promoted or produced at the expense of individual rights.

In a later article Goldman seems willing to grant that rules (such as moral policy) limiting the autonomous judgment of individuals may be beneficial for institutions (such as hospitals). He says, however, that "the burden of proof must remain with those who would defend limiting professional norms."[12] And, in fact, "deferral to such norms in morally charged contexts frequently involves the agent's sacrifice of perceived moral goods or demands, or, most regrettably, perceived moral rights."[13]

Our response is that Goldman's presupposition does not apply to our argument, for we argue not that physicians are exempt from ordinary moral obligations but, rather, that they must apply them with greater intensity because of the nature of their relationship with patients. This relationship requires greater sensitivity to need than is required in an ordinary client relationship. One may pass a sick person on the street without offering help if one is a layman; a physician can do so with far less impunity. Moral lapses such as violations of trust, when a vulnerable party is exploited or when the good of the patient is neglected, are graver than they might be in ordinary relations because of the implied or explicit covenant to care.

Second, we would argue that the Hippocratic concern for the good of the patient need not be interpreted as paternalistically as Goldman seems to have done. He also has confused beneficence with paternalism. Attacking the later, he assumes he has also "trumped" the former. As Kipnis, who is equally critical of Goldman's argument, says, "Goldman's criticism of medical ethics appears to presuppose that the well-intentioned physician is an elitist bully, committed to self-righteous lying and manipulation."[14]

Third, Goldman's assumption that social utilities must always take second place to individual rights is based in an absolutization of individualism. It would mean, for example, that production of goods potentially harmful to workers could not be tolerated. Coal production, though a social good desired by many people, would be curtailed because mining coal harms the rights of workers and burning it harms the rights of citizens to clean air. Preventive medicine's priority of a social good over individual rights would be prohibited. Efforts to block the spread of veneral disease or AIDS would not be defensible. Luban suggests, by contrast, that it may well be the case that persons have rights to basic goods (among which we would classify health and health care), and that these are "more important than the rights that must be overridden to produce them."[15]

Fourth, and even more importantly from the point of view of our thesis, the moral universe assumed by Goldman is one in which some people have roles and patients have rights. In it, universal goods are always interpreted as social utilities. This moral universe is dominated by social (utilitarian) and individual (deontological) ethical theories, without reference to the specific relationship between doctor and patient. But, as we have shown, it is not professional duty alone but the nature of the relationship itself that establishes health as the good sought in the healing relation. Further, the health sought in the relationship is not just a social utility but an individual and professional moral value. Finally, conduct on behalf of that good, as we detailed in our first chapters, passes beyond paternalism and autonomy. For these reasons any analysis of professional ethics that ignores the interactions between physician and patient is ill conceived.

RETURN TO THE RIGHTS-VERSUS-GOODS ARGUMENT

Goldman appeals to Dworkin's statement that "rights trump utilities." In this view rights are always more important than goods. Any theory of beneficence in health care is doomed to fail in favor of a theory of rights, as Dworkin proposes,[16] or a theory of patient autonomy, as Childress proposes,[17] or a number of other contractual theories of the doctor-patient relation.[18] Thus, the theory of priority of rights constitutes a second objection to our thesis on medical beneficence. It therefore calls for closer scrutiny.

Dworkin's fundamental insight is that rights are derived by persons prior to law and community. He holds that the most fundamental of these is not fairness, as Rawls thinks, but the right to an equal concern. He states, "I propose that the right to treatment as an equal must be taken to be fundamental under the liberal conception of equality. . . . I also propose that individual rights to distinct liberties must be recognized only when the fundamental right to treatment as an equal can be shown to require these rights."[19]

Dworkin's concern is to finesse two recent legal theories: positivism and economic utilitarianism. The former holds that all rights and their meanings come from law. The latter holds that rights are derived from a context of the collective welfare of individuals. Dworkin criticizes both theories as excessively rationalistic and individualistic. Searching for a theory of natural and moral rights leads Dworkin to his view that "individual rights are *political* trumps held by individuals. Individuals have rights when, for some reason, a collective goal is not a sufficient justification for denying them what they wish, as individuals, to have or to do, or not a sufficient justification for imposing some loss or injury upon them."[20] Note that rights are not viewed as absolute but as political, nurtured in and by the community.

In this view a community would be justified in promoting the good of all through preventive health measures and in penalizing those who do not look after themselves, so long as the matter were publicly debated and duly decided. Hence, Dworkin holds, "Normally it is a sufficient justification, even for an act that limits liberty, that the act is calculated to increase what the philosophers call general utility—that it is calculated to produce more over-all benefit than harm."[21] We may, for example, inconvenience a few motorists to improve traffic flow through one-way streets. Only moral or fundamental rights, such as free speech or equality, cannot be abridged. Thus, a government that professes to take rights seriously must dispense with the claim that "citizens never have a right to break its law, and it must not define citizens' rights so that these are cut off for supposed reasons of the general good."[22]

From the preceding it is clear that Dworkin does not hold a strict "rights trump goods" theory. In fact, he holds that derived, political rights may often be abridged in favor of utility. Any effort to derive an ethics for medicine from a "rights trump goods" perspective must lead to a formal analysis of a hierarchy of rights or it would not be accurate to hold that rights always trump utilities.

We think Goldman and Childress, each in his own way, are correct in insisting on the moral rights of patients to make decisions over any presumed utilities or goods of the community. However, they are incorrect in thinking that this must always be the case and that all goods are products of some sort, objective entities waiting to be put in the balance. Instead, a balance of rights and goods can be derived from the theory of beneficence we have proposed, in which rights and goods arise within the doctor-patient relation.

NORMATIVE FORCE OF BENEFICENCE

We have argued that an ethical character is imposed on the doctor-patient relation, which obligates both patients and physicians to specific moral duties that intensify common moral principles. The relationship requires an extra measure of beneficence, a heightening of common moral principles, an even more rigorous performance to specific ethical standards.[23] Most often the transcending duties will not conflict with any ordinary duties, and everything will run smoothly. But on those occasions when conflicts arise, some of these transcending duties are normative, that is, nonnegotiable *within* the relation. If the conflicts persist, the relationship must be severed to protect more fundamental rights and goods. In subsequent chapters we will focus on the characteristics of good physicians and good patients as the twin anchors of this relationshp. Here, by way of conclusion, we offer further details for some of the norms of the relationship we posed at the end of chapter 3.

CONCLUSION

The good of the patient is the most fundamental norm of the physician-patient relationship. Physicians cannot interpose other priorities, such as research goals, their personal self-interests, or institutional goals, if these conflict with the good of the patient. Similarly, patients cannot rationally refuse to comply with agreed-upon treatment or lie to their physician if these actions can be documented to harm their health.

All decisions must be mutually discussed and agreed upon unless the patient is so incapacitated by illness or accident that he or she cannot enter any agreement with the physician. In that case the physician must act as the patient's agent and presume that the patient wishes to be treated until evidence of contrary wishes surfaces. Family objections have validity only if it can be shown that they represent a prior statement of the will of the patient or represent the patient's accustomed value system. We have often heard family members say, "Mother would not want this" or "Dad would never want to go on in this condition." Chapter 13 is devoted to this topic.

Patients who rank other goods above health are certainly free to do so, but then the normal presumptions of the doctor-patient relation are modified. Physicians are under no obligation to use treatments or procedures they judge to be inadequate or injurious. In the absence of a serious violation of his or her own conscience, the physician should not abandon the patient. Rather he should provide comfort and other assistance that does not violate either the physician's or the patient's sense of values. The next chapter is devoted to a discussion of this eventuality.

The health of the community is sufficient reason to abridge individual rights if respecting those rights can be shown actually or potentially to result in direct, serious, defineable harm to the community's health. This norm is based on a recognition that human beings are simultaneously individual and social entities. No individual has a "right" to harm himself or others. To claim, for example, that an individual has a "right" to smoke, when that smoking can be shown to harm him or others, is vacuous. One could claim such a right only if stopping a person from smoking can be shown to curtail his equality of opportunity. Yet an individual does have a right to autonomy if no harm comes to others. This means that an individual has a right to strike a balance between health and pleasure. The state may curtail this right if the social consequences are too harmful. Both chapters 6 and 17 contain more complete discussions of this point.

Because both doctor and patient operate under their own ideas of the good, open and free communication must exist in the relation in order to reach consensus decisions. Neither party is justified in imposing his values on the other.

We now turn to a discussion of health and the good in the doctor-patient relation, offering a hierarchy of goods, some of which are more important than medical good. As such, acting benevolently will mean that care must be taken not to violate these goods or cherished values of the patient. Even though health is an intrinsic good of medicine, then, other goods may "trump" it when decisions are to be made about the best interests of patients.

6

The Good of the Patient

Acting for the good of the patient is the most ancient and universally acknowl-edged principle in medical ethics. It grounds ethical theories and shapes the way their principles are applied in particular cases. It is the ultimate court of appeal for the morality of medical acts. While it may be set aside for the common good, it is done so with trepidation and in only the most urgent circumstances. But so beguiling is the idea of doing good for the patient that we seldom examine closely which good, and whose good, we are serving.

Parties in a clinical decision may hold opposing views of ultimate and immediate good. Each participant is a moral agent and as such is bound to uphold and be accountable for his or her own conception of what is right and good. Making morally defensible decisions in the face of substantive differences in conceptions of patient good has therefore become one of the most urgent pro-cedural problems in medical ethics.

The problem is, of course, a subset of the deeper problems attendant on the lack of moral consensus in our society. This, in turn, is the consequence of our philosophical and theological disagreement on what constitutes The Good and the good life. A theory of good grounds every theory of morals, both general and medical. Since others are not likely to agree with our philosophical or theological definitions, we are compelled to clarify the various senses in which we may use our terms and establish an ethically defensible procedure for dealing with con-flicts when they arise.

Without such analysis of what constitutes the patient's good, emphasis usu-ally falls on the rights of patients. As we saw in chapters 2 and 3, the result can be an excessively legalistic framework for moral choice that obscures the distinctions between protecting the patient's rights and promoting the patient's good. The good of the patient must be examined independently to assure that the relationship between rights and goods is properly established.[1,2]

This chapter is an attempt to meet these two requirements—to analyze the components of patient good and to establish a procedure for handling differences in a morally defensible way. It proposes that the concept of patient good is a compound one, of which at least four senses can be discerned; that these senses are related to, but distinct from, each other; that physicians (and other health professionals) are obliged to respect each level of patient good; and that a hierarchy exists among them that determines how conflicts should be resolved. Moreover, each component can be related to the several notions of the good in Aristotle's *Ethics,* as we will show first.

Our analysis of patient good, together with related writings on the philosophy of the healing profession, constitutes our promised effort to complement and supplement the prevalent emphasis on rights- and duty-based ethical systems.[3]

PATIENT GOOD AND ARISTOTLE'S NOTION OF THE GOOD

Good is not a monolithic concept. Rather, it consists of several not entirely compatible components. This point is exemplified when the question of patient good is set in the context of contemporary views of the good and when it is contrasted with Aristotle's classical account.[4]

In a recent study, Veatch, in part following Leo Strauss, contrasts the teleology of the modern view—of contractarians and consequentialists—with that of Aristotle.[5] Modern thinkers interpret morality in terms of rights, particularly the right to define good for oneself limited only by the rights of others to do likewise. Rights then precede duties, and morality enters when the pursuit of one's own ends and interests conflicts with the same pursuit by others. In the "modern" view we cannot know what is good for the patient without knowing his or her desires. The patient's choice is good simply because she decides it. To do good for the patient, we should do the good she desires. This concept of good is most consistent with a libertarian or contractualist, antipaternalistic stance that permits the patient to choose a course even when it may seem wrong to a reasonable observer, so long as the consequences are not harmful to others.

In the classical-medieval view the good is objective and intrinsic to things that are good. These things ought to be done because they perfect one's humanity and are most fitting for humans as humans. Good, therefore, is to be determined without reference to whether the patient wants it. Freedom is thus the ability to do what one ought because one wishes to. Duty precedes rights. Indeed, rights exist because we must be unimpeded to do the good we ought to do. Patients ought not to be free to choose an evil course of action. For their good, their wishes can be overridden.

Veatch's interpretation of Aristotelian teleology may slide somewhat too easily over the controversies about precisely what Aristotle meant by the good.[6] White, for example, holds that Aristotle used good in his *Ethics* in at least three senses: (1) that which is good and desired in itself, and for which all other things are sought; (2) that which is good for a human being; or (3) that which is the aim or desire of an individual.[7] White attempts valiantly to reconcile these views in terms of *The Good,* but his efforts are not entirely convincing. It seems far more likely that Aristotle, too, had to confront the fact that humans do see The Good in at least these three ways and that these views are probably not completely reconcilable with each other.

Hardie, on the other hand, suggests that Aristotle's doctrine of The Good may be taken in two ways: the first he calls inclusive, that is, encompassing a wide variety of aims consistent with the kind of life one wants to live.[8] Humans are distinguished from other creatures as responsible planners of their own lives. Choices, therefore, are apt to be quite individual and peculiar to a personal plan of life. Hardie's second idea is of good as the dominant end. Here good is the overall plan that most fully makes a person a person, that is, the attainment of theoretical knowledge. Hardie says, "Aristotle's doctrine of the final good is a doctrine about what is 'proper' to a man, the power to reflect on his own abilities and desires and to conceive and choose for himself a satisfactory way of life."[9] This is reminiscent of Perry's general theory of value, which distinguishes humans from animals by their ability to plan ahead in accord with their interests.[10] We would like to suggest a correspondence between all four senses of patient good we have offered and the several senses in which Aristotle uses the term *good.*

Aristotle's good *simpliciter* is, of course, The Good or ultimate good. It is always in the background in clinical decisions. Even those who deny the usefulness of such a concept nonetheless have a "good of last resort," so to speak, on which they found their sense of what is morally defensible.

The second and third senses of good, as used by Aristotle (that is, the good of a particular person and the good of a human being) correspond more closely with the several senses of patient good we have discussed. The patient's interest, his idea of what is good for him and what fits his life plan, corresponds rather well with Aristotle's notion of the good as something at which people aim, the good of particular persons. Medical good, then, is the instrumental good that enables the patient to achieve his aims given the exigencies of illness.

The freedom to choose corresponds to Aristotle's third sense of the good as what is proper to a human being—someone endowed with reason: "For man therefore the life according to reason is best and pleasantest since reason more than anything else is man."[11] This passage has been interpreted as pointing to the life of contemplation but, as Hardie argues, it also points to the good of choosing, planning one's own life, and defining one's selfhood. Without freedom to choose, it is impossible to use one's reason in an effective way. Thus Aristotle says in an early work, the *Protrepticus*; "But as a rule we perform those actions well in which reason dominates."[12]

Preeminent realist that he was, Aristotle's struggle with the conception of the good probably reflects his sensitivity to any simple definition of such a compound term. The realities of clinical decisions and the trifold notion of patient good argue somewhat against those who attempt to conflate Aristotle's three conceptions into one.

Medical good, the goal of medical interest, namely, the health of the body, was for Aristotle a subsidiary good. It was a necessary condition and a means for the pursuit of the good life and the ultimate good, but was not itself ultimate.[13] Thus, in the *Rhetoric* he says, "The excellence of the body is health; that is, a condition which allows us, while keeping free from disease to have use of our bodies." But he did not think health should override other human concerns, "for many people are healthy as we are told Herodotus was, and these no one can congratulate on their health for they have to abstain from everything or nearly everything that men do."[14] With respect to physicians, he also argued that it was not abstract good, not health in general, not even the health of persons, but the health of a particular patient that was of interest to the physician.[15] Thus, the good is particularized by the body and the patient. Aristotle's assignment of health in the hierarchy of good is not very far from the position we will give to medical good in our analysis.

FOURFOLD MEANING OF THE PATIENT'S GOOD

The good of the patient is a particular kind of good that pertains to a person in a particular existential circumstance—being ill and needing the help of others to be restored to health or to cope with the assault of illness. In a general way the medical good the patient seeks is restoration of health—a return to a way of life that permits the pursuit of personal goals with a minimum of pain, discomfort, or disability. This is the end the physician promises to serve by his or her act of "profession," her promise to help with the special knowledge at her disposal. The physician thus becomes an instrument for the attainment of the good the patient seeks.

Inherent in the physician's offer to help is a promise to use her knowledge and skill for the patient's good.[16,17] This may be interpreted differently by the patient, the physician, or the patient's family. However, unless the patient is incompetent, the physician is obligated to act for the good conceived by the patient and to support the patient's goals. In this claim we opt for a more modern view of the patient's good, one in accordance with autonomy, as articulated in our conception of beneficence-in-trust. This obligation to act for the patient is limited by social constraints and public policy regarding health care. In the event those goals are morally unpalatable to the physician, she is free to withdraw from the case.

If the physician accepts the case, and as long as she maintains a relationship with the patient, she is obligated to promote four components of the patient's good: (1) ultimate good—that which constitutes the patient's ultimate standard for his or her life's choices, that which has the highest meaning for her; (2) biomedical good—that which can be achieved by medical interventions into a particular disease state; (3) the patient's perception of her own good at the particular time and circumstances of the clinical decision and how she prefers to advance her own life plan; and (4) the good of the patient as a human person capable of reasoned choices. When the patient has confused or conflicting notions of her own good, full congruence may not be possible. Nonetheless, we will argue that the physician is bound to advance each of these four senses of good to the extent possible.

Good, The Good, and the Patient's Concept of Ultimate Good

Throughout this discussion we must keep in mind the distinction between the good as perceived by the participants in clinical decisions and the ontological nature of good. This chapter cannot presume to deal adequately with the prickly question of the objectivity or nonobjectivity of the good. The point here is not whether particular interpretations of patient good are metaphysically sound. Rather, the focus is on the need for physicians, patients, and families to make decisions together, even though widely divergent interpretations do occur, and the need for dealing with conflicts, when they occur, in a morally defensible way.

But even if all participants in a clinical decision were to agree on each of the four levels in their interpretations of patient good, that would not make the decision ontologically good. One could conceive of an agreement of interpretations that would be intrinsically evil—falsification of disability or cause of death to gain compensation or insurance benefits; withholding public information of a diagnosis of plague or cholera or of a patient's homicidal intent; the practice of infanticide regarding defective infants; or euthanatizing the senile.

The good of the patient is a particular good and, like all particular goods, it is related to and shaped by the conception we hold of the notion of good and The Good. This is the first component to be examined in mapping the content of the good of the patient. What we think of the nature of good and The Good ultimately shapes all the other components.

The history of philosophical debate about the nature of The Good is too long and unsettled to be repeated here[18–21] The perennial question remains: What is the nature of The Good? Is it properly understood as one thing or many? Does it rest on some factual aspect of the nature of man or the world? Is it primarily a psychological, intuitive, or self-evident concept? Is it even susceptible to rational justification? Is the ultimate good the contemplation of truth, living in accordance with God's will, developing one's potential, wealth, honor, pleasure, power, the good of the species, or some combination of these things that adds up to "'happiness"? We need not resolve these questions to appreciate that how we answer them conditions the subsidiary notions contained in the idea of the patient's good.

The concept we hold of the ultimate good is the reference standard for all decisions, including clinical decisions. It serves to justify and define the nature and aim of moral choices. In clinical decisions some take the ultimate standard to be whatever the patient desires; others, what the physician judges to be good; and still others, conformity with philosophical, theological, or socially determined principles such as the will or law of God, the freedom of self-determination, social utility, quality of life, or the good of the species. The list is long, and the competing concepts are often incompatible.

Equally incompatible are the opposing theories of those who hold that the good is whatever humans desire or have an interest in, and those who hold the good to inhere in certain things and actions whether humans desire them or not.[22] It is not necessary to try to resolve these theoretical questions to realize that in any particular moral choice some final concept of The Good, some "good of last resort," underlies the other components of patient good. When conflicts arise in making clinical decisions with moral overtones, this final concept is the most pervasive, the least negotiable, and often the least explicit presupposition.

Biomedical Good: What Medicine Can Achieve Technically

Biomedical good encompasses the effects of medical interventions on the natural history of the disease being treated. It is the good that can be achieved by applying expert technical medical knowledge—cure, containment of disease, prevention, amelioration of symptoms, or prolongation of life. It is directly related to the physician's technical competence and is the first step in fulfilling the moral obligations of his or her promise to help. Biomedical good is the *instrumental* good the patient seeks from the physician. It is also a good internal to medicine, part of medicine's claim as a special kind of human activity. It is the good that results from the physician's craftsmanship—his capacity to make the technically correct decision and to carry it out safely, competently, and with minimal discomfort to the patient. Biomedical good is usually subsumed under the phrase *medically indicated.*

There always is an unfortunate tendency for physicians to equate biomedical good with the whole of the patient's good. We have already noted that ethicists also make this assumption. Biomedical good does not exhaust the good the physician is obliged to do. It is an essential but not sufficient component of good medicine. Two ethical errors may result from the conflation of biomedical good with the good of the patient.

The first error is to make the patient a victim of the medical imperative— to insist that if a procedure offers any physiological or therapeutic benefit then it must be done. In this view ethical medicine is limited to technically right interventions. Ethical quandaries are thus ignored since the only acknowledged good is medical good in its narrowest sense, and this is ascertained by scientific means and not by ethical discourse or analysis.

The second error is to confuse the physician's judgment of the tolerability of the quality of life that would ensue from a treatment with the medical indications for that treatment. In this view, if treatment of a defective infant results in a life without "meaningful relationships," then it is not medically indicated and should not be done. This is an unjustifiable extension of medical judgment beyond its legitimate limits. Whether a life is worth living is a value decision only the patient who must live that life can decide. Moreover, it is not a matter determinable by the capabilities of medicine qua medicine.

It is the obligation of the physician to ascertain, by the most careful method, the consequences that might ensue from a particular treatment in a particular patient. These are matters of scientific judgment proper to medicine. They are essential in helping the patient to decide if the life that ensues from treatment is worthwhile. It is the patient who must judge, with the physician's help, the kind of life he or she wishes to lead and the risks or discomfort he is willing to bear to attain the benefits medical treatment might offer.

We would argue that medical good, but *not* medicine, whould be interpreted narrowly—as that which can be ascertained scientifically and technically to be possible in altering the natural history of *this* disease in *this* person. We recognize that certain value judgments are involved, but these should be kept to a minimum and limited to scientific competence, sound clinical reasoning, and valid probabilistic statements about diagnosis, prognosis, and therapeutics. We should underline again that while biomedical good should be defined narrowly, that is not the whole of the physician's responsibility or of medicine as a practice.

The Patient's Best Interests: The Patient's Concept of His Own Good

A biomedically *or technomedically* good treatment is not automatically a good from the patient's point of view. It must be examined in the context of the patient's life situation and his or her value system. To be good in the fuller sense, the choice must square with what the patient thinks worthwhile given the circumstances and alternatives his illness forces upon him. The patient must weigh the probable medical benefits of a treatment or a no-code order (a non-resuscitation order) against the pain, disability, or loss of dignity it costs him or against some ultimate good such as his religious beliefs. When he is competent, only the patient can decide ultimately whether the quality of the life that remains is worthwhile or consistent with his belief system, or fits some plan he may have for his life. The range of satisfactions left to the sick and disabled is narrowed. But what is left may still be savored by the patient in ways the healthy person does not comprehend.

When the patient is competent, it is he who can best ascertain what is in his best interests. When he is not, his surrogates must ascertain as closely as possible what he would have chosen as in his best interests were he able to make the choice himself. Our concern must be for the person who is to live the life illness imposes, not what we think of the quality of that life.

The court in the *Shirley Dinnerstein* case, for example, asserted the legal import of the distinction between the medical decision (based on diagnosis and prognosis) and the personal decision (based on the surrogate choice by the family) of what was in their mother's best interests.[23] The medical good of a no-code order was deemed within the doctor's province; the patient's interests were placed in the hands of the family. Both were relevant for a legal decision not to resuscitate.

The patient's best interests, then, are the aims, plans, and preferences peculiar to him and chosen by him at a particular time. Any object of desire may become an object of interest for this patient at a particular time. The good in this sense is equatable with anything that is an object of interest for this patient.

Patient interest defined in this way, is necessarily subjective and relative since it is rooted in the patient's view of what is in his own best interests at a certain time and under certain circumstances. We cannot know what this is until we ask the patient. This view does not deny the possibility that some objects of interest will be bad or injurious. It is no revelation that we may know the good but do not infallibly choose it. By contrast, because someone has chosen something as good does not make it good intrinsically or instrumentally. Accepting the patient's definition of his own best interests is not the same as agreeing with them. The physician must give the most serious weight to the patient's judgment of his own interest in making decisions. Indeed, that judgment must be accorded primacy since it arises from the operation of an even more fundamental good—the human capacity to choose.

The Good of the Patient as a Person

The fourth sense of patient good is that which is most proper to being a human person. It is in a different category than the other three senses of good, each of which may be individually determined for, or by, a particular person in a particular circumstance, and may be weighted differently by different persons in different circumstances. The fourth good is the operation of the capacity to use reason to make choices, and its importance does not vary. This capacity to establish a life plan, and to select from a variety of goods those that are preferred for reasons unique and personal is a cherished and distinctive feature of human existence. Humans may not reason wisely, prudently, or correctly, but the freedom to do so is a good without which it is impossible for the mentally competent person to live a good life.

Humans who by virtue of pathological or physiological abnormalities of brain function cannot make choices (the comatose or psychotic) and infants who are not yet competent are still humans. Their choices must, perforce, be represented by others, but they must be represented nonetheless. Even though these persons cannot express their capacities to make reasoned choices, they are still beings whose nature it is to be rational. We are compelled to honor their good in this respect to the extent possible by the alternative means of surrogate or proxy decision.

Choice requires freedom, and freedom implies that some choices may be wrong or evil. Liberty and the power to choose are therefore intrinsically bound to each other. Lavelle puts it well: "For Liberty is nothing if it is not the power of choosing . . . Thus the perfect unity of the self lies in the living unity of the act which postulates and resolves this alternative . . . We can see therefore that by a kind of paradox our liberty can determine itself only by distinguishing between good and evil in the world."[24]

If we are not to violate the humanity of the patient in medical decisions, so long as the patient is competent, we must allow him or her to make his or her own choices. We cannot override those choices even if they run counter to what we think is good for the patient. To manipulate the patient's consent, to deceive or misinform her, even to do what we think is good, is to violate her good as a human being, as we saw in chapter 1. Only the patient can free us of the obligation to abide by her choices by giving us a mandate to make decisions for her if she feels emotionally or intellectually overwhelmed by the complexity of the choices. But even in the act of yielding up her prerogative, the patient exercises her freedom by choosing not to make a choice. The physician can never presume to usurp that prerogative. The freedom to choose, and to be responsible for the outcome of those choices, is the ground upon which any reasonable notion of autonomy and beneficence is built.

The good of the patient as a human is therefore a more general good than the others. It is the basis for our respect for the personal interpretations placed by particular patients in particular circumstances on biomedical good, their immediate interests, and their ultimate good. While the ultimate good is the highest good, it, too, must be freely chosen by the individual. Without freedom to choose and reject, there would be little merit in subscribing to some ultimate good, no matter how lofty.

In this regard, then, tolerance of the wide divergence of human choices and values is an essential feature of a good physician's practice. It can be enhanced by attention to the value dimension of medical theory and practice and by a thorough and continuing exploration of human experience through the arts and humanities.

Let us recapitulate the four components of the patient's good we have just outlined. In descending order of importance, they are:

1. The last or ultimate good, the telos of human life as it is perceived by the patient, his or her view of the meaning and destiny of human existence, the positions taken with reference to relationships with other men and women, the world, and God. We refer here to the good of last resort, what Tillich called an "ultimate concern," the one to which we turn for final justification of our acts if all secondary or intermediate reasons fail. That good may be contemplation of the gene pool or whatever alternatives humans might choose.

2. The good of the patient as a human person, the good that is grounded in his capacity as a human being to reason, and therefore to choose, and to express those choices in speech with other humans who can also reason and speak. Freedom to choose is the irreducible condition of functioning as a human distinct from other species. Its violation results in an enslavement of the humanity of one person to another. Hence, these first two values clearly supersede the next two values, which follow.

3. The patient's best interests, that is, the patient's subjective assessment of the quality of life the intervention might produce, and whether or not he deems

it consistent with his life plan, goals, and aims. This life plan will be highly personal. The choices that might advance it may well run counter to biomedical good or what the physician thinks is a good life for the patient. The problem of quality of life is important enough to devote a complete chapter to its discussion, which we will do in chapter 7.

4. Medical, biomedical, or clinical good—the good that can be achieved by medical interventions into a particular disease state. This good is usually expressed by medical indications—the statement of what can be achieved based on strictly scientific and technical assessments. These judgments should not be confused with judgments from another person's perspective about the quality of life that would result.

In every human decision, and especially in clinical decisions, these four senses of the good are intermingled. The configuration of choices we make at each of these levels and the way we relate one to the other in large part defines us as persons. Each level must be understood and respected. When they are in conflict, or are interpreted differently by the parties making medical decisions, some hierarchical order must be established among them. Without such an order decision making is paralyzed or, worse still, results in the imposition of one person's choices on another.

To acknowledge that these four levels of good can differ among interacting humans is not to accede to the idea that all choices are equally valid logically, epistemologically, or metaphysically. No capitulation is being made here to moral relativism or emotivism. There are morally good and bad choices at each level, and these distinctions must not be abandoned. They must be recognized, and morally sound procedures established, so that each element of patient good is adequately promoted in the face of potential conflicts among the interacting parties. Such procedures might consist of a requirement that physicians negotiate all treatment with their patients, a consequence of our earlier reflections on beneficence-in-trust and one that, at least in the view of Abram, may help reduce the malpractice crisis.[25] Another requirement might be the establishment of ethical hospital policies that would govern the hierarchy of values involved in the physician-patient relationship, especially if such policies were to be developed by committees that included laypersons, as do some hospital ethics committees.[26]

Of course, the ethics of procedures can be clearly differentiated from those of substantive issues. Further, the good of the patient must also be related to social good, not only because individuals are social beings, but also because the freedoms we enjoy are delimited by the common good, by social roles and duties, and by the law and entitlements of others. Some implications of social realities for the beneficence model have already been established in chapter 2, in which we discussed the perils of autonomy and the nature of a democracy. More clinically relevant consequences will be discussed in the final section of this book, especially in those chapters dealing with incompetent patients, the role of the family in clinical decisions, and the physician as gatekeeper. Nonetheless, a brief sketch of resolutions using the hierarchy of values follows so that more difficult problems can be compared with the normal set of priorities based on beneficence-in-trust.

PROCEDURES FOR RECONCILING CONFLICTS

We have concentrated on the meaning of the patient's good because this is the raison d'être of all clinical medicine. But as the cumulative effects of individual medical decisions alter the world's demography, and as high technology consumes an ever-larger percentage of its resources, the other good things a society seeks come more and more into conflict with the good of individual patients. Already the economic and social costs of prolonging the lives of many aged and disabled patients are intruding themselves into clinical decisions. Medicine's more vocal critics are taking it to task for overemphasizing the good of individual patients while neglecting the good of society. As a result, the principles of social and distributive justice are increasingly invoked as relevant within clinical decisions.

Consequently, physicians are being pressured to assume the role of monitors of the social and economic good of society, yet patient good and social good often come into conflict. How consistent is a concern for social good with the traditional ethical commitment of physicians to do everything to advance the interests and medical good of their patients?

These sorts of questions underscore the need not only for a more explicit analysis of the points of conflict stemming from a beneficence model but also for their resolution, if possible. The resolution, in turn, requires establishment of some sort of hierarchial order among the various competing goods if decisions are to be made on any principled basis. We attempt some resolutions in the latter part of this book as examples of how the beneficence-in-trust approach can contribute concrete action plans regarding incompetent patients, the role of the family in medical decisions, and the physician as gatekeeper.

For now we will propose a system of priorities among goods as part of the theory of beneficence we advance. This system aims more precisely at establishing a "normal" template for the resolution of conflicts of goods between doctors and patients, although some attention is paid to social values as well. Social values are not the main point, however. Making clinical decisions with moral implications necessitates some ranking of goods because they can often come into conflict. After we propose an objective procedure for resolving conflicts, we will examine more closely the hierarchial relationship that should occur among the four senses of patient good.

As we mentioned, conflicts between good things can be resolved ethically only by recourse to some rational organizing principle. The principle we propose is beneficence-in-trust. The way the principles of beneficence, nonmaleficence, justice, truth-telling, and promise-keeping are applied in clinical situations is linked to the interpretation one makes of the good of the patient. The order we choose is based on a preferential option to trust the perceptions of patients about their own good unless, of course, there is reason to suspect that perception. The hierarchial order we propose might differ from other proposals on the basis of the following variables: how patient good is defined; what preferential option is chosen (for example, paternalists might prefer physician judgment first); and what goods are considered objectively to be more important than others in one's philosophy of medicine.

There are at least two ways of looking at the structure of relative weights to be assigned competing goods. The first is procedural and the second is metaethical. The first, which receives the most attention in medical ethics and the philosophy of medicine, is an approach based on establishing a process in the absence of any perceivable consensus about the relative importance of various values or goods. Nonetheless, the procedure itself implies a certain preferential option, which in turn reveals a metaethical bias. Jonsen, Siegler, and Winslade, for example, employ a guide for making decisions about patients that reveals just such a bias since preferences are based on the nearness to or distance from the patient's own wishes. These authors note in *Clinical Ethics* something we have also emphasized. Conflicts of goods (which they call *principles*) occur in the clinical setting and the practice of medicine; the need for some external priority principle is therefore evident. Which values and goods, which levels— as we have described them—should receive more weight than others in such decisions? These authors rank the ethical importance of the values in the relationship in the following order: first, patient preference; second, medical indications; third, quality of life; and fourth, external factors.[27] We suggest a slightly modified order below.

Procedural Scheme

Clear Directives from the Patient

The first presumption in any normal state of affairs must be for the patient's preferences. But not all preferences are appropriate. Hence, we introduce the word *clear*, by which we do mean neither those preferences with which others most likely would agree nor those that other reasonable persons find important. Rather, we mean those preferences based quite consistently on the patient's own values. Hence, if a patient dying of cancer had consistently refused resuscitation but during his or her last hours begs to be put on a respirator because of difficulty in breathing, the preference or wish can no longer be seen as part of a clearly related value plan. The physician may order the respirator for other reasons— such as making the patient comfortable—even if the patient is now incompetent by virtue of hypoxia or hyperapnea.

Negotiated Values of the Patient

Normally, these interests are articulated by the patient in the preceding step, although they are often distinct from current judgments the patient may make.

The example of the patient who requests a respirator during his last hours is a case in point. The best interests he has revealed in previous dialogue with the physician and his family are to not prolong his dying process. His current request for a respirator, then, is clearly a preference, but simultaneously, and less clearly, is also in his best interests. It is this sort of problem that makes simplistic appeals to living wills and patient preferences so dangerous in the ethics of medicine. The physician might choose to deny the patient's request in this case, then, on the basis of the patient's best interests as the patient had previously and consistently portrayed them.

Sometimes, too, the physician must judge what is in the patient's best interest, in the absence of current wishes. We will examine this point in more detail in the last section of the book, but by placing this value second in our procedural scheme, we underscore the importance of the physician acting in the best interests of his or her patient. This implies, and this point is exceptionally important, that the physician knows the patient's own hierarchy of values, either through the ways in which the patient has chosen or employed values in the past or through the process of negotiation we earlier discussed as essential to the fiduciary relation in medicine itself. Many physicians are strangers to patients in our modern system of health care. This makes it even more important for such physicians to have in hand some objective document outlining patient values (an expanded version of the living will, perhaps) or otherwise ascertaining the patient's value system. Most often this is done with the patient or family in an informal way. We will say more about this in our chapters on incompetent patients and family decision making.

Proxy Judgments

The judgments of proxies constitute the next step in a methodology for resolving dilemmas in decision making. If the patient cannot express preferences and has not left a statement or otherwise conveyed a judgment of his or her best interests, then the physician must turn to proxies to express the wishes of the patient. As the court noted in the *Conroy* case, patients, once incompetent, do not lose their right to make decisions about their health care. Instead, proxies must speak for their values. The normal presumption is, of course, that the proxy is trustworthy. The reason this step is not second in our scheme is that previously expressed wishes are not always a good guide for making current decisions. This is true not only because people change their minds in new circumstances but because people cannot foresee all situations to be covered by their wishes. That is why we prefer to discuss the best interests of patients as they perceive them, thus gaining a more comprehensive set of values about life than the focus on individual clinical decisions (for example, the use of a respirator if I am dying) or preferences. Here it is of less value to respect trustworthy presumptions conveyed by proxies than the patient's own established values, precisely because these are still presumptions. In our scheme then, although important, presumptions are less certain to represent actual patient decision making than are negotiated values the patient might make with the physician in the step described above. Of course, if the patient had never participated in such negotiation, the proxy recommendation about preferences should be taken into account.

Hospital Ethics Committee Resolution

If for some reason the physician and patient (or the patient's proxy) cannot reach a mutually agreed upon resolution, we propose that the hospital ethics committee structure be used. In this scheme an effort to resolve conflicts should always be made first at the bedside before involving the hospital ethics committee. Nevertheless, conflicts involving the patient, physician, hospital, and legal system sometimes occur (as they did in many court cases such as *Conroy, Brophy, Bartling,* and *Bouvia*). In this event an attempt to reach a consensus should be made prior to an appeal to the legal system.[28] Clear directions from the patient or clearly documented negotiated values always take precedence over this step unless such preferences or negotiations threaten important values of the profession and/ or the hospital itself. As we argued in our previous work, health care teams and institutions themselves are subject to moral commitments.[29]

These conflicts need to be resolved as closely as possible to these persons affected by the decision. It is important to note that proxy revelation of patient value systems or patient preferences need not always be respected if, in the physician's judgment, there is some obvious conflict of interest or if this revelation is not in accord with the patient's own negotiation about best interests that might have taken place independently and prior to the necessity for a proxy. Although this is not normally the case, it is a good example of the kind of disagreement that might later arise between a proxy and the physician and should be considered by the hospital ethics committee for possible resolution.

Legal System Appeal

Either because of the nature of the conflicts or the lack of social unanimity about certain procedures, or because no conflict resolution could be made locally, appeal must be made finally to the legal system. In some instances, as in child abuse cases, a guardian will be appointed by the court. In others the court itself will attempt to resolve the medical decision. In such instances courts proceed according to the steps laid down in the *Conroy* case already discussed.

Metaethical Scheme

A second way of resolving conflicts is to appeal to an objective scheme based on a philosophy of medicine. This is a metaethical scheme because it establishes priorities on the basis of philosophical criteria of good. Ethics alone cannot justify such a hierarchy. Instead, it requires the philosophy of medicine's insights into fundamental principles of the discipline itself. In other words, this scheme is based not so much on the patient's preferences as on the ranking of the goods themselves (one of the goods being the patient's preferences, of course). The ranking we proposed in this chapter is maintained: first, the patient's ultimate good; second, the good of a patient as a human person; third, the patient's particular good; and fourth, biomedical good.

Physicians would employ this hierarchy in decision making by guiding the negotiation session with patients along these lines, and by exercising the preferential option for patient decision making in the absence of suspicions about its inauthenticity. In this way at least the first two steps of the procedural hierarchy would be guided by as clear an exposition as possible of the patient's own values, to be placed in each of the four categories of the metaphysical scheme. Further, decisions to disagree with the patient's hierarchy (and possibly withdraw from the case) would be based on the content of this objective structure of values. How would that negotiation proceed?

The Good of Last Resort

Some of us clearly organize our lives around one good that is the highest good, traditionally the *summum bonum*. For those who reject this idea, we refer simply to the "good of last resort"—that good to which we tend to return whenever we are forced to make choices between competing goods, the one good we tend to place above others. For the religious person, perhaps, the highest good is accommodation to the will or law of the Creator. For the nonreligious it may be the greatest pleasure, the least harm, the greatest utility, enlightened self-interest, the good of the least advantaged person in a society, the absolute autonomy of patients to choose, or the survival of the species. As we pointed out, we need only accept that there is de facto such a good for all who attempt to make rational choices. Even pluralistic intuitionists must base their intuitions on a final good in this sense.

Clearly, the ultimate good, or the good of last resort, will take precedence over other forms of patient good. Paternalism, strong or weak, with respect to a patient's choice of ultimate good is morally offensive. The ultimate good is the starting point of a person's moral reasoning, his or her first act of intellectual faith, so to speak. If she is competent, the patient's wish must be respected over medical good, and over the physician's, society's, the family's, or the law's construal of ultimate good. The patient may abandon or subjugate her conception of ultimate good to her more immediate personal interests, but others may not do so for her.

When a patient does abandon her highest value—for example, when a Jehovah's Witness agrees to accept a blood transfusion in order to save her life—what should be the physician's response? Should the physician not accept this betrayal by the patient and instead insist on the patient's ultimate values? The answer is no. The physician would respect the patient, according to the first step of the procedural scheme already proposed. Thus, since the value of the ultimate good is held by the patient (and not necessarily by the physician), when the patient abandons it, the physician is under no obligation to remind the patient of its importance.

Most persons, however, seek out medical care from those with whom they agree on the ultimate principles so that, if they do continue to choose such beliefs, their choice will not be belittled. While the refusal of therapy for religious reasons is often discussed in the medical ethics literature, a different sort of denial of the ultimate good principle is not. That is the problem of overtreatment. If the physician, hospital, and patient all share a common faith or are members of a religious belief system that stresses the finitude of life and its transcendent purpose, then overtreatment of dying patients can constitute a betrayal of the ultimate good held by the patient (and, in this instance, by the physician and hospital).

When conflicts occur in decisions involving human life—such as no-code orders, discontinuing life-support measures, artificial insemination, or abortion—they often involve disagreements about the ultimate good and are therefore reconcilable with great difficulty, if at all. Under such circumstances the physician-patient relationship should be respectfully and courteously discontinued since neither physician nor patient can in good conscience compromise a profound belief system.

The Good of the Patient

The next good, in order of priority, is the good of the patient as a human person, the freedom to make his or her own decisions. To place medical good or the quality of life ahead of freedom to choose is to rob the patient of his humanity. The physician, instead, has the obligation to enhance the patient's competence in every way—treating pathophysiological disturbances of brain function, freely providing accurate information needed to make choices, and refraining from coercion or deception even to overcome resistance to needed treatments.

The once-competent person who at the time of decision is comatose, psychotic, or otherwise unable to reason and choose does not lose claim as a human being to have his interests respected. This is a major legal point raised by recent cases and given both summary and impetus by the *Conroy* court. We turn, therefore, to surrogates or proxies who can act on behalf of those interests. Presumably, the surrogate knows the patient or is close to his cultural or ethical values system. If the physician does know the patient's values, he or she becomes the patient's advocate and supersedes decisions made by proxies only on the basis of presumptions. These surrogate's choices should approximate what the patient would have wanted were he able to express his choice.

In the difficult situation in which there is doubt about the capability or good intention of the surrogate, the physician must attend to the good of the patient. This may require resorting to the hospital ethics committee or the courts if the physician thinks the surrogate's decision is not in the patient's interests (recall the fourth and fifth steps of the procedural scheme). Under these circumstances, at least the patient's legal rights can be protected and the intentions of both the surrogate and the physician examined a little more objectively, recognizing always that a legal decision may not necessarily be a morally correct one. We take up the problem of incompetent patients and surrogate decision making in the last section of the book.

The Particular Good

The third step in the objective scheme is the patient's own perception of the particular good of the moment. The difference between this and the previous step, then, is the difference between laying down a life plan or system of values and making an individual choice or preference about treatment. Step 3 decisions by patients are most often ones in which the values in steps 1 and 2 are reconciled with an action plan (steps 3 and 4). In this third step the patient must grapple with quality-of-life judgments. As we will show in chapter 7, these judgments are made by clinicians when trying to adjust treatment to outcomes based on medical indications. But patients themselves also make such judgments, for example, when a patient chooses between several medical options for breast cancer. This choice often rests on a balance of many values. When physicians make quality-of-life judgments, they should, as a rule, do so based on the patient's own assessment of that quality of life. When this becomes impossible the appeals to the procedural steps enumerated above should be made.

Another example of the particular good option is the following. A patient develops hypertension. His physician recommends a threefold treatment plan: First, salt will be eliminated from the diet. Second, the patient will go on a diet to reduce his weight by thirty pounds. Third, medication will be used to bring down the blood pressure immediately. If the patient rejects the latter step (a medically indicated one) because of the possibly intolerable side effects of impotence, should the physician continue to accept this patient? Should the physician drop the patient? This is an interesting question because the patient has not completely rejected the recommended treatment plan, but only the most intolerable and yet effective step in the plan. The presumption is that the physician has explained in detail the statistical dangers in which the patient places himself by not bringing down his malignant hypertension. Clearly, the patient has made a quality-of-life judgment that differs from the one the physician might make for him or from the medical indications (biomedical good) appropriate for his care. We suggest that the physician might, indeed, have to withdraw from the case if he or she judged that the patient's care would be severely compromised by such a step.

A third example of the patient's own formation of individual decisions (this time through a proxy) comes from follow-up discussions in the press about William Schroeder's course after receiving a Jarvik VII artificial heart at the Humana Heart Institute in Louisville. Recall that Schroeder's course was complicated by a series of strokes, now thought caused by clots that formed along the valves in the artificial heart and then traveled to the brain. When asked about whether "Bill" would have wanted to try the artificial heart had he known ahead of time that he would be alive in a chronic debilitated state, Schroeder's surgeon, Dr. William De Vries, replied that there was no question in his mind that Schroeder would have wanted to live. When further pressed about whether this was true, given Schroeder's compromised mental status, De Vries claimed that there was no doubt about it.[30] Yet, a few months later, another interview took place, this time with Schroeder's wife. She was asked the same sorts of questions and, in response, argued that her husband never would have wanted the artificial heart if he had known what a burden this compromised state would have put on his family and how he could not have enjoyed life.[31]

In this exchange it is clear that Schroeder's wife, as a proxy, was expressing a step 2 value system (a life plan or system of values) that demonstrated the kinds of values Schroeder had about his family and his own life. From these she was postulating that her husband's individual judgment about quality of life would be that the operation was not worth it. The reason for this is that he saw the operation as an either/ or proposition. Either he would die almost immediately of heart disease or he would have a chance to live (albeit dependent on machines). According to his wife, he did not foresee an in-between state, a state of being neither dead nor alive, as a consequence of his decision. If he had, she argues, he would have made a quality-of-life judgment and foregone the transplant.

According to the hierarchy of values we have proposed, the patient's own quality-of-life judgments take precedence over judgments made about the patient by others, but are themselves superseded by (or, more often, are derived from) their life plan or system of values accounted for in step 2.

Biomedical Good

The final objective criterion for treatment is biomedical good. In the absence of any other supervening value, the biomedical good as we have defined it should be the basis of physician decision making for the best interests of patients. We have explained how this value is important in a beneficence-in-trust theory of medicine. By now the following should be clear: First physicians and patients most often assume this good as the basis for the exchange in the doctor-patient relationship. Second, neither physicians nor patients are totally bound by biomedical goods in establishing the negotiated good to govern that relationship. However, the patient drives any changes in the good governing the relation. For example, it is not proper for physicians to establish as their primary duty the fostering of religious convictions in their patients (step 1). But if a patient negotiates respect for his or her religious values, the physician is bound to respect these values when making decisions. Third, it is clear that physicians are always bound to present the biomedical good to the patient as their recommendation in the absence of any supervening values of the patient or negotiated values in the relationship.

Obviously, not all the moral obligations that derive from this scheme of patient good are spelled out here. Health professionals, health care institutions, ministers, families, and friends—all who participate in decisions that affect those who are ill—must take into account the many dimensions of patient good. In the best decisions the four senses we have outlined should be closely congruent. When they are not, the differences should be spelled out as clearly as possible and negotiated with honesty and sensitivity. This is an instance in which the quality of the personal relationships and the character traits of the interacting parties will often be more important than rules or procedures.

The hierarchical orders we have suggested have implications for the way the common principles of medical ethics are applied. This is pertinent for each of the several varieties of paternalism.[32] The physician who is a strong paternalist, for example, places biomedical good above other senses of patient good. For him, the patient's perceptions of his own immediate or ultimate good, his freedom as a person to make his own immediate or ultimate good, and his freedom as a person to make his own choices are not primary concerns. For some strong paternalists, technomedical good justifies withholding or manipulating information or breaking promises.* Even the use of deceit or force might be rationalized to assure compliance with what is medically indicated.

Conversely, the libertarian typically places personal autonomy at the head of the list of what is good for the patient. A Rawlsean contractarian would opt for the good of the least advantaged member of society, though a Hobbesian would not be so inclined.

CONCLUSION

Everyone who participates in a clinical decision justifies actions as being on behalf of the patient's good. We have tried in this chapter to show how complex a concept the patient's good actually is. First of all, it involves definitions of good that are derived from diverse and sometimes competing philosophies, theologies, and personal constructions. Secondly, it is composed of at least four factors, which we have discussed, and, in the final section, justified their ranking by appeal to a set of metaethical assumptions that guided the hierarchial order. In addition, as we have noted, the patient's good is often negotiated, and when it cannot be, a procedural scheme is necessary for resolving troublesome problems. Some of these problems occur when personal and professional values conflict with social values. We only noted these for further discussion later. In addition, we will use our procedural scheme in the chapter on the role of the family in medical decisions as an example of how it might be employed to resolve difficulties and contribute to the development of institutional and even national policies.

We have suggested that a proper analysis of the patient's good will make for more ethically sound physician-patient relationship and a clearer interpretation of the usual principles of medical ethics. Since conflicts between the patient's perception of good at this moment (the quality-of-life problem) and biomedical good are one major way in which goods conflict in the clinical setting, we devote the next chapter to examining this conflict.

---

*Note that other reasons exist to break promises or withhold the truth, such as concern for the health or well-being of others; these reasons are not based on biomedical good.[18]

7

Quality-of-Life Judgments
and Medical Indications

A traditional duty of physicians has been to act in the best interests of their patients.[1] A direct line can be traced from the Hippocratic corpus to the present day regarding this duty. It is the legacy of beneficence so important over the centuries to patients and to physicians.[2] As long as physicians could reasonably assume that the best interests of patients could be equated with the preservation of life, acting beneficently created few problems. Beneficence meant making right and good clinical decisions. A right or correct clinical decision was one corresponding to the best medical standards. A good clinical decision was a right decision made in line with important ethical values of the patient, physician, institution, and society.[3]

In this chapter we examine the challenges medical progress poses for traditional assumptions about beneficence. These problems raise the question of quality-of-life judgments. Such judgments presume that the best interests of others match our perceptions of their interests. We proceed as follows: First, three challenges to beneficence are presented; then the need for quality-of-life judgments is sketched; and, finally, concerns about making quality-of-life judgments are presented, along with responses in the form of axioms. What will emerge is the view that medical indications, properly understood, form the only valid basis for quality-of-life judgments.

THREE CHALLENGES TO BENEFICENCE

Three major challenges to the traditional duty of acting in the best interests of patients have arisen in today's medical practice. These challenges make right and good clinical decisions far more difficult to accomplish than in the past.

The first of these challenges is the technological imperative. Dramatic advances in medical technology have tempted physicians to misidentify what is best for the patient with the newest available technique. Oftentimes the technological imperative leads physicians to equate the patient's best interests solely with the medically indicated course of action in such cases, rather than with values the patient may profess.* As we shall see, this equation is sometimes valid, but only under certain very limited circumstances. It is not valid as a general rule for patients who are competent to articulate their own values.

The second challenge comes from the consequences of technological interventions in the case of technological difficulties. Physicians can now keep patients alive far beyond the plane of normal effective and cognitive existence. This is especially true regarding patients who suffer chronic illnesses such as diabetes or cardiovascular disease. In effect, the possibilities in medical technology foster the equation of the best interest of patients with the preservation of life. More often than not, such identification works well, particularly if that is the value chosen by the patient in the clinical relationship. But it may not work well for an elderly, hypertensive, post-myocardial infarct patient who has suffered a massive bilateral stroke and is in a permanent vegetative state on a respirator.

The difficulty lies in judging where to draw the line between preserving life and permitting death. Either everyone in similar circumstances should be treated equally—for example, all those who suffer a bilateral stroke should remain on a respirator—or some discrimination should be made on a case-by-case basis. As soon as the best interest of a person is no longer the preservation of life, then physicians (and family members) are forced into the ethical quandary of making judgments about treatment when life is so fragile and death so imminent that "letting the patient die" may be in his or her best interest.

The third challenge comes from another quarter. This is the patient rights movement, which permits, among many other things, the patient to decide what is in his or her best interest by making preferences about care known to the physician. Such autonomous decision making seems to conflict with the duty to act in the best interest of patients when the medically prescribed course of action is refused by the patient. A number of court decisions have legally reinforced the philosophy of autonomous decision making by ruling that patients may elect to remove themselves from life-supporting technology, even over the objections of their physicians and the hospitals that care for them.

The shape of these decisions goes back at least as far as the case of Karen Ann Quinlan. In that decision the Supreme Court of New Jersey declared that Quinlan's previous wishes regarding the respirator were made known to family and friends, and that her parents acted correctly in insisting that these wishes be followed.[4] More recently, the same court dealt with the case of Claire C. Conroy, an elderly, senile patient in a nursing home. Although the issue in this case was

---

*This is one of the central theses of the present volume.

a feeding tube, the decision was similar: that the patient, although now incompetent, did not lose her right to make decisions about her care, which were now to be expressed by her nephew.[5] Many physicians are concerned about the extensive procedures established by states such as New Jersey to ensure that decisions about treatment discontinuance be monitored. Nevins noted recently that, despite a favorable response from citizens about the decision the Supreme Court made in the *Conroy* case, physicians and laypersons in the know about the requirements that the court instituted are far less approving. In New Jersey nursing homes, for example, patients may no longer die without a feeding tube in place. Once a decision has been made to forego life support or withdraw it altogether (even if this decision is based on the patient's own preferences), it appears that a cumbersome process must be initiated whereby an ombudsman office, as well as two additional physicians, must be consulted.[6]

The first two challenges restrict traditional beneficent decision making by turning such decisions into paternalism, acting in the best interests of patients without their consent or in the absence of their consent. The last challenge restricts clinical decision making by promoting patient autonomy and state bureaucracy over the traditional role of the physician. All three present a challenge to physicians to become much more sophisticated about ethical and legal norms governing such decisions than they might have been in the past. Under what circumstances, then, can beneficent decisions be made? And how are these different from decisions based simply on a medically indicated course of action?

QUALITY-OF-LIFE JUDGMENTS

So-called quality-of-life decisions must be approached with the greatest caution. Inadvertently, they influence clinical decisions when the life the patient is living or the dying he or she is undergoing is so unaffected by medical treatments as to make continued intervention futile or seriously burdensome to the patient. We respect the value of every human life, however it may be afflicted by illness, disability, pain, or suffering. In this sense life itself, independently of the person who lives it, has a quality that must be respected.

But when the end of life is near and inevitable, and when attempts to reverse the dying process are futile, the continuance of life no longer has any possibility of satisfaction for the patient. Indeed, to continue may be an affront to the dignity of the patient, representing a kind of therapeutic belligerence. Under these stringent conditions the quality of that patient's life is wanting—*not* his value as a human being. We ought to allow the natural history of the disease to take its course.

We would warn against quality-of-life judgments outside of these stringent conditions. We object to any facile judgments about the quality of another person's life. Because of the tendency to confuse quality of life with value of life, we prefer not to use the term except in the strictly limited sense defined here.

Assessment of the benefits and harms of continued treatment may be the only way left in some cases to avoid inflicting harm or cruelty on patients.[7] Those who agree that such judgments are indeed necessary normally suggest that the criterion be strictly defined. An example might be that it is possible to withhold treatment if it would cause too much suffering or if the patient were in a permanent vegetative state. It is often difficult to ascertain whether or not a patient may be in extremis. Even with the best diagnostic and therapeutic modalities, it may be hard to predict how long patients may survive with or without treatment. It is always difficult to decide whether any given intervention may create or prolong suffering.

One would think that these factors would limit the use of quality-of-life judgments in physicians' decisions. Yet, as Pearlman and Jonsen have determined, of 205 physicians surveyed about a hypothetical case involving a decision to intubate, 37 percent used quality-of-life judgments in some way. Fortynine percent of those who decided not to withhold mechanical ventilation justified their decision by an appeal to quality of life, while 87 percent of those who chose not to intubate appealed to quality-of-life factors. One major conclusion of the study was that the notion of quality of life has no obvious meaning. As the authors point out, "It is not clear to which empirical states the term refers, nor is it manifest how any particular person will evaluate those states."[8]

As Pearlman and Speer argue, our views about the quality of life of others are notoriously off the mark.[9] A lack of guidelines, as Hilfiker illustrates, renders these judgments subjective, capricious, and, in the end, guilt ridden.[10] This is especially true with regard to chronically ill cardiovascular patients,[11,12] incapacitated elderly patients,[13] and other hopelessly ill patients or those who cannot speak for themselves.[14]

In the face of uncertainties about either status or values, therapeutic actions are equally uncertain. Some, like Hilfiker, confess that they "do nothing" or "go slowly" in such circumstances. This is one way to allow "nature to take its course." This approach is contested by those who say that it lacks the respect for human life that is essential to the very nature of medicine. Still others base their decision on "positive outcomes"—that is, specific organ system progress— although even this approach fails near the end of a person's life. Reluctance to make quality-of-life judgments, as mentioned, stems either from uncertainty about the patient's own value system. Society's values are also involved in the latter uncertainty. Let us examine these in more detail.

Clinical Status Uncertainty

While most physicians are comfortable with making medical judgments about a person's current status, given the technological advances of modern medicine, it is difficult to make prognostic judgments about some patients. For instance, a patient who suffers from a terminal form of congestive heart failure may present to the hospital for the sixth time in a year, with decreasing intervals between admissions. Although the prognosis is dim, one cannot judge at present that this will be the last admission, or that current interventions only serve to prolong suffering or to violate the ethical axiom that it is wrong to prolong the dying process.

If a patient makes his or her own value judgments, she can inform the physician about preferences regarding certain treatments that will prolong life. Thus, personal evaluation is the primary means by which to make judgments about initiating or discontinuing treatment. The physician's judgment about interventions can therefore be based on the patient's desires with respect to the panoply of techniques and medications available.

When the patient becomes incompetent, previously expressed wishes become very important. These could have been articulated to the managing physician or to family members. If both agree that certain interventions were ruled out by the patient, then the proper course of action is to respect those wishes.

Even when the clinical status of the person is indeed hopeless, the family or patient may wish to continue "at all costs." Most physicians find this event less difficult than others, and act on the basis of such wishes. However, when health policy itself determines that certain conditions do not warrant reimbursable treatment (for example, when the patient does not improve after ten days on the respirator), physicians face a difficult dilemma. Their allegiance to the patient is challenged. This allegiance is transformed into public policy at great risk.

Another dilemma occurs when a patient formerly expressed no explicit wishes about treatment and later becomes incompetent to do so. The clinical status of the patient is either chronic (in this case a chronic vegetative state or chronic senility that would render the patient incompetent) or hopeless (irreversible, terminal illness is present as well). Great variability then occurs in treatment plans. Some physicians appeal to quality of life as an assessment of the hopelessness of the condition. They move the chronic or hopeless patient into the category of "dying" and they apply to the patient the ethical axiom of not prolonging dying through further interventions. The only aim of therapy, therefore, is keeping the patient comfortable. Other physicians appeal to the technological imperative already mentioned, or identify the patient's best interests with certain interventions that may or may not improve the status of a particular organ system. For example, the oxygen output may improve although the patient, in any real sense, has not regained an effective and cognitive human life.

The latter course should be carefully examined. It assumes that medical indications are simply objective standards to which one can appeal without question. In fact, medical indications are an amalgam of objective data, accepted medical practices, and the interpretation of the fit between the patient's condition and the intervention.

Value Uncertainty

In making these judgments the physician must not only evaluate the medical status of the patient. He or she must also examine the personal status of that patient. This means that the patient's values must also be taken into account in making clinical decisions about care.

The situation is clear, as it was above, when the patient can make his or her own evaluation of quality of life. It is not so clear when that preference has not been clearly expressed (through discussion with family, a living will, an advanced directive, or negotiation with the physician). A good example might be an elderly heart patient, transferred from a nursing home, who is without a family. How should one proceed?

If no reliable evidence of past or present wishes can be evoked, the physician, acting in the best interests of the patient, must base treatment decisions on medical indications. This does not mean it is best to treat in all cases, however.

First, the medical indications should be examined from the point of view of the whole person rather than just an individual organ system. The question to be answered is: Will this treatment be not only effective but beneficent to this patient? Will it provide care, amelioration of symptoms, and comfort?

In answering this question the clinical status, probable values of the patient, and the best-case outcome of the intervention are all measured against the prognosis. The *Conroy* court added to this consideration the requirement that the treatment not be cruel or create further suffering. While the court was concerned about withdrawing treatment, this requirement would also logically seem to apply to contemplated interventions.

At no time, of course, should the physician judge that a patient's life is not worth living, or that a patient has no value in society. It is both morally and legally inappropriate to measure the value of a person in society and use this as the basis of treatment decisions. Medicine must always be free to treat without regard to the cause of the disease or the economic status of the patient who suffers. The proper role of social values in health care is to delineate the standards of access to health care. If a public policy decision has been made to limit the use of respirators or kidney dialysis—as it has been in England, for example— then that limitation, applied equally to all patients, could be a legitimate consideration in a treatment decision about an incompetent patient.

TWO AXIOMS

Two axioms regarding quality-of-life judgments are presented as a way of summarizing this discussion. First, the physician is not obligated to prolong aggressive treatment if there is virtually no likelihood of benefit from the intervention. This axiom is based on a judgment that it would be cruel to continue treatment in light of medical indications alone. It differs from Ramsey's proposal regarding medical indications. Ramsey would have all treatments that are medically indicated instituted on the grounds that no one has an absolute right to refuse treatment. Thus, his medical indications policy seems to propose that even competent patients cannot refuse therapy if such refusal would lead to death.[16] Adoption of Ramsey's policy would lead to overriding autonomously made patient decisions about care. Further, his policy would seem to require that any medically indicated treatment that would prolong life would have to be ordered. Both features are ill-advised—the first because it would lead to a violation of privacy, the right to be left alone, and the legally approved right to make health decisions; and the second because it would lead to disproportionate use of medical care, even when hopeless outcomes are inevitable. Thus, some subjective judgment of "reasonableness" or the proportion between benefit and burden is required.[17] But this judgment should be related to the next axiom as well.

According to the second axiom, the physician is not obligated to continue treatment if such treatment requires the use of severely depleted health care resources and the benefits of the proposed intervention are not significant. This axiom is based on a theory of justice in which each person is treated the same unless there is some morally relevant difference among them.[18] The morally relevant difference in cases covered by this axiom would be the lack of any truly significant benefit for the person taken as a whole. That is why we would most likely offer heart surgery to someone who could resume a decent quality of life after the surgery but not to someone who would gain little or nothing from such surgery. It is not that the latter person is less "valued" than the former by society or by medicine. Rather, the latter person suffers from an impairment for which we have no effective treatment.

It is best to argue that patients deserve the degree of treatment that would bring about a restoration of comfort and decent function. This does not mean that, to justify an intervention, the patient would have to regain a function in society long ago lost to them because of their chronic disease. Instead, it means that the results of the current intervention should be compared with the state of function the patient enjoyed even while under the influence of the chronic or hopeless disease. Additionally, the fact that the patient has already had a chance to compete for the goods and services of society should also be taken into account.

Very expensive treatments that lead to minuscule benefits are therefore proscribed by this axiom. In this regard, not every treatment that appeals to the age criterion is questionable if age is regarded as an indicator of medical suitability. Nor is the use of age as one medical indication entirely inappropriate, since we all age and will all be treated equally in this respect in the future.[19] In this sense, then, the ratio between treatment and benefit shrinks as one reaches old age and faces chronic illness.

8

The Good Patient

Much of medical ethics, appropriately, deals with the obligations of physicians to patients. However, there is also a set of obligations that binds the other partners in the medical transaction—the patients and, by extension, their families, surrogates, or proxies, where appropriate. In this chapter we examine the responsibilities of the good patient, complementing our next chapter, which deals with the characteristics of the good physician.

In our theory of beneficence in health care, professionals and patients have moral obligations to each other. The normative character of the relationship permits us to speak of what *ought* to be done in making clinical decisions. But we must not overlook the qualities of character, the kinds of persons patients and physicians ought to *be*.[1] A fuller critique of the kinds of institutions and societies most conducive to a morally valid healing relationship is also needed. This is beyond the scope of this volume, but its significance for the content of this chapter cannot be ignored.

PATIENT ROLE EXPECTATIONS

A number of studies have investigated what physicians, nurses, and patients themselves consider a good patient. Not surprisingly, the professional's view of a good patient is one who "is kind," "is willing to suffer," "is affable," "is not irritable," "asks for help," "obeys orders," "does not complain," and the like. These descriptions obviously flow from a particular model of health care in which patients are seen as passive and suppliant participants in actions done to them.

This is how our culture expects sick persons to behave. The sick role, as Talcott Parsons and others have shown, is defined by one's particular culture.[2] Insofar as a patient conforms to this role, he or she is branded a good or bad patient. In this way, being sick, which itself is a morally neutral state, becomes morally tinctured.

There are significant differences in descriptions of the sick in various cultures. For example, in the United States, Glazer reported that along with obeying doctor's orders, a good patient was most frequently identified as one who tries to help himself.[3] In the United States the obedience—self-help axis is a dominant feature of the physician-patient relationship. Bhanumathi compared descriptions of a good patient in the United States with those in India; she showed that respondents from the United States identified and emphasized autonomy and independence, while those from India chose passivity and dependence. She theorized that this was because of the traditional family structures and interdependence among family members that characterize Indian life today.[4]

Several studies give evidence of disagreement between professional and lay descriptions of the good patient. These, too, are culturally dependent. Thus, in a Czech study, a relatively stable idea of a good patient emerged in which laypersons and health professionals consistently agreed within the context of socialized medicine.[5] This study contrasts with one conducted a decade earlier by Freidson in the United States.[6] In Freidson's study there was less agreement among doctors and patients about the qualities of a good patient than in the Czech study. Inaccurate and even unethical descriptions of a good patient also occur, as in the reported tendency among physicians to consider all beautiful persons good patients.[7] Further, evidence exists that "good" patients (as perceived by doctors) may not actually tell health professionals the truth about their progress or compliance.[8] Some studies identify a good patient with one who keeps coming back, thus enhancing one's practice;[9] or as one who utilizes a health center more frequently than others.[10]

The health care system in the United States is frequently criticized for depersonalizing patients in favor of efficiency.[11] As a result, people are treated as nonpersons or objects,[12] or are denied even ordinary civilities such as being introduced to the doctor.[13] At the root of these and like criticisms is the fact, as Lorber puts it, that "doctors and nurses deliberately limit the communication of information to patients to prevent their work routines from constantly being interrupted with questions or to mask their shortcomings and failures from the scrutiny of clients who are living where they work."[14] All of these views tend to make the patient an object of the doctor's many ministrations, to be processed but not to respond to, or participate in, that processing.

Lorber's study confirms that, while professionals and patients may sometimes agree on the characteristics of the good patient, they may still differ in the degree to which the role should be played. Clashes occur, therefore, not only over the characteristics of the good patient, but also over the degree to which a particular patient may wish to conform to one or another likeness.

The beneficence model we have advanced requires a balance of decision making in the doctor-patient relationship. Just as there are qualities that define a good doctor, there are also qualities that define a good patient. These qualities will sometimes correspond with those identified in the aforementioned studies and sometimes not. We seek to ground our definition in the nature of the relationship between one who is ill and one who professes to help. It is the fundamental nature of the human experience of being ill and being helped, rather than roles defined by social, economic, or political considerations, that, for us, defines the good patient and the good physician.

Before setting forth our view of the qualities of a good patient, we shall examine four currently proposed health care models—the business, contractual, covenant, and preventive models. These lead to contrasting views of the good patient, and differ in many respects from the theory we propose. Thus, we will describe our theory as a fifth model, one based in beneficence, which incorporates the best of the other four models without their weaknesses.

MODELS OF HEALTH CARE

Childress and Siegler have studied, rather thoroughly, how different systems of metaphors and models about medicine condition they way practitioners view their roles and their medical-moral principles.[15] We shall use a similar idea to explore how different models can lead to competing views about the moral principles involved in health care, and about which virtues we might expect the good patient, or good physician, to exhibit.

Model A: Business Relation

In the business model medicine is viewed as a commodity transaction not too different from buying an auto or taking it to a mechanic. This model is often used by hospital administrators, health planners, and economists. The services

Table 1. Models of Health Care

Model	Nature of Health Care	Nature of Relationship	Professional's Obligation
A. *Business*	Commodity	Buyer and seller	Commitment, Skill
B. *Contractual*	Service	Contracting equals	Supply specific service
C. *Covenant*	Obligation	Sacred trust	Commitment to life
D. *Preventive*	Life-style	Unilateral option	Not applicable
E. *Beneficent*	Negotiated good	Trust (fiduciary bond)	Act for good of patient

of hospitals, for example, might be described as "product lines" to be judged by their economic viability, market demand, or income-producing capabilities. The relation between physician and patient is most often described as that between a professional and his or her client. The professional, in this view, is defined explicitly or implicitly as anyone highly skilled and highly paid compared with others in society. Since health care is a commodity to be bought and sold in the marketplace, the patient becomes a purchaser of services. The purchaser or client bargains for the commodity, exchanges funds for services, and possesses the rights and duties usually accorded a consumer in a free-market economy.

With this model the good patient is one who contributes to a health economy by paying bills on time, by being a repeat customer for preferred services, by complying with instructions for which one has paid a fee, and by knowing how to make a good purchase. One either follows the advice in which he or she has invested or changes his purveyor.

The ethical obligations of doctor and patient to each other are minimal. The doctor must provide a "good product" and stand behind it; the patient must pay for the expert service he or she received. Presumably, the physician can set any fee he or she feels the market will bear; the patient will pay whatever health care is "worth" to him. The guiding mores are, for the patient, caveat emptor; for the physician, providing a good product, not because it is morally owed to the patient but because it is good for business to have a reputation for good service. This is close to the preservation of one's reputation which preoccupied the Greek physician.[16]

The ethical obligations of the business model are simply the ethics of good business and good consumerism—a good product on the one hand, and enough knowledge and skill on the patient's part to shop wisely. The ethical obligations of physicians and patients to each other are legal in nature, and failures in the transaction are tested in court—civil or criminal, depending on the nature of the dissatisfaction. The Federal Trade Commission (FTC) would thus regulate these commodity transactions and would assure that no restraint of trade is practiced, even if it is advantageous to the consumer.

Model B: Contractual Relation

The contractual model grows in popularity daily, largely because so many people want to protect themselves against the physician's paternalism or economic self-interest. We already discussed this model in some detail in chapter 4. It extends the commodity transaction model by calling for a contract to formalize the business relationship. It has all the characteristics of the business model but is explicit about what is required of transacting parties. It is a translation into the medical realm of the Lockean notion of the autonomous individual.

The contractual model regards both doctor and patient as equal partners in a commodity transaction. Veatch, for example, has proposed a tri–level contractual model for the decisions to be made in health care.[17] Veatch, and Freidson as well, emphasize that professionals have often been privileged and powerful persons. Freidson, in particular, has written on the damaging nature of professionalism through which persons come to acquire power and class interest not commensurate with their overall knowledge and sensitivity to human nature.[18] In order to counteract that kind of power and the paternalism it breeds, patients are seen as autonomous entities. Those who propose the contractual model hope to close the power gap between a powerful class of health professionals and their vulnerable patients.

A person is autonomous who can make independent judgments about ideas and conduct and carry these judgments out in private and in public. An autonomous entity is capable of self-definition and self-determination. Health care in this model becomes an item of negotiation between these powerful and autonomous entities. This model requires that the patient be viewed as someone capable of making up his or her own mind about his or her health affairs. Such a model obscures the clinical realities of serious illness and disease, and their impact on persons.[19] As a matter of fact, the contractual model often presumes more autonomy than patients can muster, a point of criticism we raised in chapter 1.

The contractual model seeks to limit the region of trust between doctor and patient. It presumes that the range of services must be anticipated in detail; it does not allow for sufficient unexpected events. If it tries to anticipate the unexpected by phrases like "as needed" or "as indicated," it defeats itself because it thus widens the range of events over which trust must operate.

The contractual model mitigates somewhat the principle of caveat emptor, but it generates the same minimalist ethical requirements, largely those based in law rather than morality per se. It tends to interpret justice, truth-telling, promise-keeping, nonmaleficence, and beneficence as terms of legal rights and duties, rather than trust in the virtue or character of the participants in the transaction.

Finally, the contractual model assumes that the contracting parties are really equal. It is difficult to envision someone who is ill, in need of help, worried, and anxious as equal in the face of the physician's knowledge and skill. Can a sick person negotiate a contract in any real sense?

Model C: Covenant

The third model describes the relationship between physicians and patients as a covenant. This grounds the relationship in the sacred, with its rich connotations of trust and obligation. It is therefore the opposite of the idea of a legal contract or commodity transaction. It is difficult to communicate the complete idea of a covenant in secular terms, but its meaning must be better grasped if we are to move beyond the inadequacies of commodity and contractual theories of medicine.

Three of our most distinguished ethicists—Veatch, Ramsey, and May—have contributed to the elucidation of the concept of covenant. In his more recent work, Veatch has moved away from the contractual model and closer to the covenant model. He seems concerned to avoid the reduction of medical ethics to legalisms, to mitigate somewhat his insistence on patient autonomy, and to emphasize more fully the social responsibility of the physician. In his view, physicians and patients enter covenantal relationships so that physicians may be partially exempt from social duties in order to pay particular attention to the needs of their own patients.[20] Veatch thus modifies the contractual model by leaning more heavily on a theory of social justice in health care and the physician's professional obligations within that theory.

May's use of a covenant model is quite different. His model, like Ramsey's, rests on an explicitly religious foundation. Through it, medical exchanges are elements of interpersonal relations in which both physician and patient are locked in the human condition. Illness is part of the struggle to be human. In both May's and Ramsey's views, the professional is committed to help the patient because the patient is a fellow participant in life, facing what is universally a part of the human condition. The act of profession is therefore an act of commitment to life stemming from the nature of the condition rather than from a contract for a commodity or service, or from a theory of social obligation.

But May's concern differs from Ramsey's in at least one important respect.[21] May wants to reject any form of medical paternalism in this model. In this he shares Veatch's respect for patient autonomy. In fact, beneficence itself strikes him as a theory of medicine that emphasizes the *receiving* nature of care by the physician.[22] Although we think this is an entirely accurate description of a relationship of need found in medicine, we do agree with May that it should not be interpreted as an occasion for paternalism. Thus, for him, a covenant model preserves a fundamental equality of persons, the professional and the patient, who both give and receive from one another.

Ramsey's later work on ethics "at the edges of life" contrasts with interpretations of the covenant model emphasizing patient autonomy and the equality of physician and patient in the relation. In his view the patient, like the physician, is obliged to act on behalf of life. Hence, physicians may override patient decisions if the latter somehow fail to respect the value of life itself. Ramsey argues that patients do not have an absolute right to refuse therapy because they have an obligation to preserve their own lives.[23] Thus, a patient cannot be viewed solely as an absolutely autonomous entity. As a human being the patient has profound obligations toward life and toward health.

The virtuous or good patient, in this interpretation, is one who fulfills his or her deontological duties toward life and toward other persons. Ramsey errs in identifying health with virtue itself. Health is good, as we have argued thus far, but it is not necessarily a moral good, or at least not a moral good of such weight that it must be given priority over all other values in a person's life (see our previous discussion of the hierarchy of goods in chapter 6).

Model D: Preventive (No Relation)

In the fourth model medicine is not defined as a relationship at all. Instead, any action to preserve health is considered to be part of medicine. Whitbeck has proposed that jogging and weight lifting are just as much medical acts as going to the doctor.[24] In this view, then, professionals become social engineers of a sort. They engineer society to protect as many "healths" as possible by establishing social policies and encouraging walking, playing racquetball, brushing teeth, and so on. This model rejects the idea of legal contracts, covenants, or other bonding mechanisms. Through contracts, people are responsible for their own health; they would approach health professionals only when they need information they themselves cannot find or help they cannot obtain elsewhere. Many major diseases are partially caused by aberrant life-styles. Since the latter are often within the total control of the person, there is some substance to this model.

Each of these models has strengths and weaknesses. The business model is important in an age of diminishing resources, but it fails to touch on the more sensitive and profound aspects of the medical relationship found in the covenant model. The contractual model properly delineates some of the duties of physician and patient, but only within the context of the legal aspect of the medical relationship and without much attention to the clinical realities of illness. By contrast, the covenant model describes some of the more profound aspects of the medical relation experienced by practitioners and patients alike. In Ramsey's version it totally equates the "health" of the patient as a moral obligation with its medical definition. The preventive model extends the valid point of self-help to the entire medical enterprise. To do so is to fall victim to a misapplication of analogical reasoning. The preventive model fails to take into account the very real state of dependence, vulnerability, and limitations on freedom that the loss of health entails.

Model E: Beneficent

In our view the beneficent model best incorporates the good points of the foregoing models without their failings. It offers, we believe, a clearer delineation of the mutual obligations of physicians and patients with respect to the good of health.

In the beneficent model, the physician and patient are joined through the bond of a particular kind of human need. The need is that of the patient for healing. The physician or health professional is one who responds and who makes right (correct) and good (moral) judgments with, and on behalf of, the patient.[25] Health is a negotiable good, one that may move up and down a hierarchy of values as perceived by the patient. It is not an absolute and overriding value.

In this model the patient is one who suffers a need he or she cannot fulfill unaided. The patient needs help from another who can provide relief for that need. The patient is dependent on another human being who "professes" to be able to help. The bond of need creates an obligation in the professional to act on behalf of the patient. The health professions are ordained by society primarily for this purpose and not for entrepreneurship, since the patient's need exists independently of the ability to pay. To pay is not a requirement, except acciden-tally.[26] Further, the bond of need, which May wishes to de-emphasize, is not an occasion for confusing the good of the patient with paternalism. As we have argued, beneficence includes respect for patient wishes.

A patient in the state of "wounded humanity" that illness implies is not, however, capable of totally free, informed consent or autonomy. Disease and accidents disrupt the personal integration normally enjoyed by the patient and in its place, cause anxiety, fear, pain, dread, and a host of other impediments to acts that are full, free, and voluntary. Most of all, the patient is vulnerable since he or she must seek help and is dependent on the competence and empathy of the health professional. This vulnerability and dependence create obligations that the virtuous physician voluntarily assumes, which were spelled out in chap-ter 7. We now turn to a similar task with respect to patients.

VIRTUES OF A GOOD PATIENT

At this point in our argument, we have left behind the initial descriptions of a good patient in terms of compliance and self-help. By definition, a patient is one who "suffers," who bears a disability, who is in need of help. To this definition we have added the qualities of vulnerability, disruption, and dependency. To the degree that the patient is able to maintain some basic form of human free-dom (as opposed to being comatose or incapable of decisions or action), that patient may be described as good who (1) is scrupulous about telling the truth; (2) is compliant about the agreed-upon steps to recovery or palliation; (3) avoids manipulation of other patients and the health professionals who care for him or her (if hospitalized); and (4) trusts to the extent that the bond with the physician is not lightly regarded or violated.

We have grounded the source of the physician's obligations in the special nature of illness as a human experience, the needs it generates for help, and the voluntary promise of the physician—his or her act of "profession" to help. What grounds the moral obligations of patients? What are the characteristics of the good patient?

First of all, the patient, like the physician, has all the obligations of any human being in moral relationship with others—truth-telling, promise-keeping, beneficence, justice, and the like. In addition, because a patient is one who is ill, these obligations are identified by the special nature of the healing relationship. That relationship assumes that the patient is honestly seeking assistance, that once he and the physician have negotiated a morally valid consent, he will coop-erate with the physician. As Katz has so commandingly argued, the doctor-patient relation in our time requires sustained dialogue without duplicity.[27]

Both doctor and patient share a common goal—the restoration of health. The patient is assumed not to enter the relationship for personal gain—for example, to deceive the physician for some ulterior purpose such as gaining workmen's compensation insurance, luring the physician into grounds for malpractice, falsifying a work record, or feigning symptoms to get a prescription for narcotics or psychopharmaceuticals. The patient's very act of seeking help elicits in the physician a sincere promise to help, and that promise, in turn, imposes on the patient the obligation to enter the relationship with honest motives and to cooperate in the agreed-upon decisions and actions. The patient must trust the physician; the physician must trust the patient. While the patient is eminently exploitable, so, too, in a sense, is the physician because he is expected by view of his professional and social role to practice a certain degree of self-effacement and restraint of his own self-interests.

In general, fewer obligations are demanded of the patient than the physician. One reason is that the patient's motives for entering the relationship are more limited than the physician's. The major "profit" he seeks is to be made well, or to be helped to make himself well (except in the instances mentioned above). Where the leverage in an unequal relationship is so firmly on one side— the physician's—the moral obligations must be weightier on that side, too.

Patients, then, must relate to physicians in all of the virtuous ways that govern human interrelationships and social conduct. Under this obligation would fall the usual matters of justice, such as paying the physician on time, keeping promises and appointments, acting with civility and courtesy, and the like. Insofar as patients are patients, four virtues are particularly required: truthfulness, probity (compliance), tolerance of others, and trust. Of these, only the first two are essential to the medical process; the last are helpful but not absolutely required to bring about the healing end of medicine.

Truthfulness

Patients must tell the truth so that accurate history taking and workup may proceed. This obligation is built into the medical relationship and is independent of a contractual relationship. If healing is a moral good, then the qualities needed to attain it are virtues as well, if one defines virtue as Aristotle did (a good operative habit). The patient must be truthful about his or her present condition or complaint, and his values and obligations that will influence his choices of alternatives. The last is necessary so that the physician may act as the patient's advocate and also understand where their values might differ. If this is not done, physicians are caught by surprise when patients disagree with their recommendations by rejecting what is medically indicated. Everything possible should be done to elicit patient response regarding values about life, quality of life, and the like, in any serious medical decision.

Interestingly, the AMA Code of Ethics of 1847 recognized the importance of the patient's truthfulness. It states that, after the duty to seek help from physicians, "patients should faithfully and unreservedly communicate to their physician the supposed cause of their disease ... A patient should never be afraid of thus making his physician his friend and advisor."[28]

It is from this need for disclosure of the truth that the corresponding duty of physicians to preserve confidentiality is derived. The AMA code of 1847 puts it this way: Patients "should always bear in mind that a medical man is under the strongest obligations of secrecy."[29] As Renshaw has noted in this regard:

> A physician is often told much more than a priest in the brief time of the confessional. Unlike an African witchdoctor [sic], who is expected with the aid of special bones to discover hidden causes of a silent patient's problems, our patients are expected to tell in great detail every aspect of their own history plus that of consanguineous relatives. Openness, honesty, accuracy, and concise detail are all hallmarks of "good" patients.[30]

Patients can err against the virtue of truthfulness out of anxiety, pride, or mistrust of the physician. A patient may deny having previous chest pains, only later telling the physician that he or she was afraid of facing the serious possibility of heart disease or cancer. This fear can lead to unconscious distortion of, or deliberate lies about, the patient's history. The history may also be deliberately distorted if psychological or financial advantages might accrue from illness.

Probity

We have chosen the word *probity* instead of *compliance* to avoid negative, paternalistic connotations. *Compliance* is, of course, a perfectly decent word if cited in conjunction with a mutually agreed-upon plan. The important point here is that the patient, having formed a relationship with the physician regarding healing, having truthfully conveyed information about his or her condition and history, and having agreed to a specific treatment plan, must concentrate on doing her part to achieve her own healing.

The virtue of probity covers not only traditionally understood compliance in negotiated treatment plans but also elements of forthrightness if the plan has not been followed. Otherwise, the plan might be adjusted needlessly, with greater risks and fewer benefits to the patient. In fact, deception about compliance tends artificially, but nonetheless forcefully, to impose the patient's own values on the physician by covert manipulation.[31]

Justice and Tolerance

In this age of malpractice suits, justice is too often interpreted as winning a suit against the physician. Yet justice must also recognize what is owed the physician—protection of his reputation and his personal life from the emotional and fiscal damage of capricious suits. Even if lawyers are willing to enter suit or calculate that a "case" can be made that will result in some award, however just the claim may be, the patient has a responsibility to act justly. Capricious or unwarranted suits, fraudulent information provided to insurance companies, falsified statements requested of physicians, and a host of other practices that would in health be rejected are often encouraged during illness. Clearly, a virtuous patient will recognize the moral indefensibility of such actions.

We have argued strenuously in this book and elsewhere for the physician's understanding of and tolerance for the patient's values and the impact of illness on the patient as a person. But tolerance of some degree is also owed the physician. Patients need to comprehend the inherent limitations of medicine to cure all diseases, somatic and psychic. There is also the inherent fallibility of medicine, so well outlined by Gorovitz and MacIntyre.[32] Certain procedures and treatments carry irreducible risks, discomforts, and mortality. Not all congenital anomalies, or even birth injuries, are the result of the obstetrician's negligence. Getting well, especially through the use of complicated technical maneuvers, is impossible without some risks. This is why informed consent is so essential. But informed consent, when properly obtained, carries with it the obligation for tolerance when the predicted, or unexpected, mishap occurs.

Further, patients must appreciate that some of the hostility to physicians, nurses, and hospitals is really hostility against the misfortune or seeming unfairness of illness itself. Also, the physiological accompaniments of illness may well modify the patient's usual personality or stress responses.

Recognition of all these factors imposes some obligation for the good patient to exercise the virtue of tolerance for the physician and other health professionals. Failure to exhibit this virtue is often at the basis of capricious or unwarranted malpractice suits. We are not pleading here for amnesty for the negligent physician; rather, we plead for a realistic comprehension on the part of patients that illness, the risks of getting well, and the personality changes that accompany illness impose a moral obligation of tolerance on the responsible patient.

The virtue of tolerance should extend to relationships with fellow patients in hospitals or clinics as well. Patients can damage their fellow patients' confidence in their own physicians by unduly frightening them about their disease or baselessly questioning the competence of other doctors. They should not impose their own views about clinical decisions on other patients. Often, because of physical proximity or because they are suffering from the same disease, hospitalized patients can have a more powerful effect on each other than can physicians. It goes without saying, too, that respect for other patients in such matters as smoking, noise, television, and number of visitors, is an important obligation of hospitalized patients.

Trust

Trust cannot be fully excluded in the physician-patient relationship. The patient ultimately needs to place some confidence in the relationship with the physician if therapeutic aims are to be carried out. We do not mean that the patient must explicitly subjugate all his or her judgments to those of the physician. Rather, enough mutual trust should exist that the patient feels free to disagree, to discuss value changes in the course of the disease, and to adjust expectations throughout the duration of the illness. An element of gratitude and friendship is part of this virtue as well. Seneca wondered why it was, for example, that he felt such a strong friendship for his physician, who had put himself out in Seneca's cause.[33] He answered the question in much the same way as the AMA 1847 code directs: "A patient should, after his recovery, entertain a just and enduring sense of the value of the services rendered him by his physician; for these are of such a character, that no mere pecuniary acknowledgement can repay or cancel them."[34]

We emphasize the need for trust because, no matter how tightly a contract may be written or a covenant explicated, medical care depends upon a continuous series of judgment calls and competent acts that cannot be predicted precisely in advance. There are many small "moments of truth" in which the good physician, trying to meet his obligations and promises to the patient, must take action based on his or her own judgment of what he interprets to be the best interests of his patient. The virtuous physician is one who in these moments approximates most closely the best interests of the patient. The good patient is the one who recognizes his or her own responsibility to facilitate his own healing by enabling the physician to act in his best interests, and by judging the result with justice and tolerance.

The virtues just described form the basis of a fundamentally and sound relationship with the physician in which healing may take place. Truthfulness and probity are absolutely essential to effective healing. Justice, tolerance, and trust enhance this relation without detracting from it. They are not absolutely necessary for the healing relationship to occur, yet they can often impede it if absent and enhance it measurably when present.

Certain characteristics are expected of patients, depending on the model one accepts of the physician-patient relationship. We have argued that beneficence is the best model in which to view the patient's role, and the virtues that make for a good patient are intrinsic to this model. We will now turn to a discussion of the good physician.

9

The Good Physician

Consider From what noble seed you spring: You were created not to live like beasts, but for pursuit of virtue and of
knowledge.

Dante, *Inferno*

Benevolence, wishing the patient's good, and beneficence, doing the patient's good, arise from several sources—for example, respecting inherent rights, recognizing duties and obligations, or being a person who habitually desires and does the right and good thing. While the emphasis today is almost wholly on the respect of rights and duties, ultimately, the physician's character, or to put it another way, his virtue, is the ultimate guarantee that the patient's good will be respected.

In this chapter we examine the virtues of the physician as a person and as a physician, and their relationship to the good of the patient. We shall try to show that a virtue-based ethics must be linked to a rights-and-duty–based ethics if we are to provide maximal protection of all dimensions of the patient's good. Like it or not, in our democratic society, even the guarantees of rights-and-duty–based ethics are dependent upon the physician's character. Some review of the concept of virtue as it pertains to the healing relationship is therefore in order.

THE CONCEPT OF VIRTUE

In the opening pages of *Dominations and Powers,* Santayana asserts that "human society owes all its warmth and vitality to the intrinsic virtue in its members" and that the virtues, therefore, are always "hovering silently" over his pages.[1] And, indeed, the virtues have always hovered over any theory of morals. They give credibility to the moral life; they assure that it will be something more than a catalogue of rights, duties, and rules. Virtue adds that extra "cubit" that lifts ethics out of its legalisms and into the higher reaches of moral sensitivity.

Yet, as MacIntyre's brilliant treatise so ably attests, virtue-based ethics has, since the Enlightenment, become a dubious enterprise.[2] We have lost a consensus. There is no vantage point from which to judge what is right and good. Virtue becomes confused with conformity to the conventions of social and institutional life. The accolades go to those who get along and get ahead. Without agreeing on the nature of the good, moreover, we can hardly know what a "disposition" to do the right and good may mean.

These uncertainties force us to rely on ethical systems built upon specific rights, duties, and the application of rules and principles. Their concreteness seems to promise protection against capricious and antiethical interpretations of vice and virtue. But that concreteness turns to illusion once we try to agree on what is the right and good thing to do in a given circumstance.

Despite the erosion of the concept of virtue, it remains an inescapable reality in moral transactions. We know there are people we can trust to temper self-interest, to be honest, truthful, faithful, and just, even in the face of the omnipresent evil. Sadly, we also know that there are others who cannot be trusted habitually to act well. We may not be virtuous ourselves, we may even sneer at the folly of the virtuous man in our age, yet we can recognize him nonetheless. As Marcus Aurelius said, "No thing delights as much as the examples of the virtues when they are exhibited in the morals of those who live with us and present themselves in abundance as far as possible. Wherefore we must keep these before us."[3]

And, in fact, the virtues are again being brought before us in the resurgence of interest in virtue-based ethics.[4-17] For the most part the resurgence is based in a reexamination, clarification, and refurbishment of the classical-medieval concept of virtue. The contemporary reappraisal is not an abnegation of rights-and-duty–based ethics but a recognition that, rights and duties notwithstanding, their moral effectiveness still turns on the disposition and character traits of our fellow men and women.

This is preeminently true in medical ethics, where the vulnerability and dependence of the sick person force him or her to trust not just in her rights, but in the kind of person the physician is. In illness, when we are most exploitable, we are also most dependent upon the kind of person who will intend, and do, the right and the good thing because he or she cannot really do otherwise. The variability with which this trust is honored and, at times, its outright violation account for the current decline in the moral credibility of the medical profession. They account, too, for the trend toward asserting patients' rights more forcefully in contractual as opposed to covenantal models of the physician-patient relationship.

THE CLASSICAL-MEDIEVAL CONCEPT OF VIRTUE

What is virtue? What are the virtues? Are they one or many? Can they be taught? These are still the fundamental, first-order questions for any virtue-based ethical theory. And, like so many of the perennial philosophical questions, they were first examined in an orderly way in the Platonic dialogues. In the early dialogues Socrates raises them with his characteristic to-and-from probing. Given his circumambulation of definitions and the difficulties of translating from ancient languages, Socrates' precise meanings remain somewhat problematic.

Most commentators, however, focus on his equilibration, in the *Meno, Protagoras,* and *Gorgias,* of virtue *(aretē)* with knowledge *(epistēmē)*.[18-21] Virtue is here synonymous with excellence in living the good life. This excellence depends upon knowledge of good, evil, and self. It is not specialized knowledge directed to any one activity, but rather to living one's whole life well. It must, like an art, be perfected through practice. The individual virtues—courage, justice, temperance, wisdom, and piety—order life toward excellence. But they, too, depend on knowledge, so that, in this view, vice is the result primarily of ignorance.

How much of this intellectualistic definition of virtue is Socrates' and how much Plato's is debatable. In the later dialogues, the *Laws* and the *Republic,* more attention is given to justice as a central virtue and to proper ordering of the state.[22] Wisdom is still a virtue, but for the statesman it is knowledge of what is good not just for the individual good life but the good of the whole state. The aim of laws should be virtue, but the chief virtue is wisdom, so that wisdom is the knowledge that "presides" over justice.[23]

In the *Republic,* still exploring definitions, Plato draws the analogy of virtue with bodily health: "Virtue then as it seems would be a certain health, beauty and good condition of a soul, and vice a sickness, ugliness and weakness."[24] He likens virtue to the order and balance between the parts of the body that characterize health. For Socrates that ordering results from intellectual perfection of the art of living a good life. Plato, as Aristotle pointed out, paid more attention than Socrates to the nonrational elements in human life. Virtue, for Aristotle, is as much a matter of disposition to act in the right way as it is a desire for the good, arising from knowledge of the good.

Aristotle reacted to Socrates' overintellectualization of virtue. He devoted large portions of the *Nicomachean Ethics* to his concept of virtue. His own work, Aristotle said, "does not aim at theoretical knowledge like the others (for we are inquiring not in order to know what virtue is, but in order to become good, since otherwise our inquiry would have been of no use), we must examine the nature of actions, namely, how we ought to do them."[25] He does not reject the role of intellect; he judges it a proper part of virtue but not its whole. Thus, he emphasizes that virtue is also concerned with feelings and actions: "Just acts are pleasant to the lover of justice and in general virtuous acts to the lover of virtue."[26]

But virtue is not just feeling. It is of two kinds: intellectual and moral: "Intellectual virtue in the main owes both its birth and growth to teaching (for which reasons it requires experience and time) while moral virtue comes about as a result of habit, whence also its name *ethikē* is one that is formed by a slight variation from the word *ethos* (habit)."[27] Virtue is not simply a passion or a function, but a "state of character."[28] Virtue is that state of character "which makes a man good and which makes him do his own work well."[29]

But states of character must be in accord with the "right rule." Hence, the intellectual virtues play a part in making a man virtuous. Practical wisdom is that aspect of intellect that enables a man to direct his life to its chief good. The right rule is reached, as Ross says, "by the deliberative analysis of the practically wise man and telling him that the end of human life is to be best attained by certain actions which are intermediate between extremes. Obedience to such a rule is moral virtue."[30]

Aristotle's doctrine of the mean, and his divisions and subdivisions of the intellectual and moral virtues are too complex to engage us here.[31] What is significant for the present discussion is the balance Aristotle strikes between moral virtue and reason, feelings, dispositions, and right action. These are Aristotle's modifications and extensions of the Socratic notion of virtue.

Aristotle also made more explicit the Socratic orientation of virtue to ends. Thus, "Every virtue or excellence both brings into good condition the thing of which it is the excellence and makes the work of that thing to be done well."[32] The end of virtue for both Socrates and Aristotle is the good life. What constitutes the good life is, for both of them, fulfillment of the potentiality of human nature.

Aristotle summarizes the essential elements that distinguish the virtuous man: "In the first place he must have knowledge, secondly he must choose the acts and choose them for their own sakes, and thirdly his actions must proceed from a firm and unchangeable character."[33] This combination of character, knowledge, and deliberate choice makes for a virtuous person. Actions themselves are virtuous when they emanate from just such a person. For Aristotle, then, virtue resides not only in the act or in the knowledge of virtue, but the act itself must also be done virtuously, as a virtuous man would do it. "But as a condition of the possession of the virtues knowledge has little or no weight, while the other conditions count not for a little, but for everything."[34] Nor does virtue reside in the act itself.

Saint Thomas Aquinas' treatment of the virtues is best understood in the context of his total enterprise, which was to reconcile, emend, and amend the ancient philosophers through the revealed truths of the Christian experience. Precisely to what extent his emphasis on the cardinal virtues coincides with or departs from Aristotle is difficult to say. Aquinas, too, had to surmount the problem of trying to apprehend the nuances of words in an ancient language no longer in daily use. MacIntyre calls him a "marginal figure," not representing the general opinion of the virtues extant in his time. He does, however, recognize that Aquinas' interpretation of the *Nicomachean Ethics* "has never been bettered."[35]

For Aristotle the intellectual and moral virtues are requisite for the full development of man's natural capacities. But, for Aquinas, man's natural end is itself insufficient because man has a spiritual destiny that transcends the merely natural. Man is destined to union with God. To this end, both natural and supernatural virtues are needed, and these can be known only through revelation. For the Christian the perfection of the natural virtues is not sufficient.[36]

Like Aristotle, Aquinas thinks virtue is grounded in good habits, in dispositions to do the right and good thing, but always in association with right reason. Thus, he says, "It belongs to human virtue to make a good man and his work according to reason."[37] And, "Through virtue man is ordered to the utmost limit of his capacity."[38] It is a condition of the perfection of human life. Or, said another way, "Virtue is called the limit of potentiality . . . because it causes an inclination to the highest act which a faculty can perform."[39]

Virtues for Aquinas are habits and dispositions that enable a man to reason well (the intellectual virtues) and to act in accordance with a right reason (moral virtues)—*recta ration factilium.*[40] These two kinds of virtue can be independent of each other, but in the virtuous man, who strives for the perfection of his human potentiality, they are joined. And they are joined most firmly in one virtue from which the others derive—prudence, the standard of right willing and acting, the form and mold for the other virtues.

Among modern commentators, Pieper has most clearly expounded Aquinas' teaching on prudence and the other cardinal virtues.[41] Without attempting to restate that teaching here, suffice it to say that for Aquinas all virtue is necessarily prudent, acting in accord with right reason in conformity with the reality of things. This is not prudence in the pejorative modern sense of caution, timidty, rationalized cowardice, cunning, or casuistic deviousness. Rather, it is the analogue of Aristotle's wisdom, the capacity and disposition to will and act rightly in particular, practical, and uncertain circumstances. As such, prudence informs, measures, guides, shapes, and generates the other virtues by inclining us to choose good means to good ends for man.

The postmedieval transformations of the classical concepts were many: Rousseau opposed virtue to society; for Shaftesbury virtue lay in the pursuit of public interest; Hutcheson and Hume identified it with a "moral sense"; to Montaigne virtue was "an innocence, accidental and fortuitious"; for Descartes, strength of soul; for Malebranche, love of order; for Spinoza, the soul directing itself by a universal and clear idea; Mandeville paradoxically defended the utility of the vices. MacIntyre delineates, with a wealth of detail, the continuing emotivist and intuitionist trends of philosophies of virtue since the Enlightenment.

In the last several years, the classical concept has been reexamined by a growing number of moral philosophers. They have underscored such things as the difference in meanings of the words *aretē* in Greek, *virtutes* in Latin, and *virtue* in English; the distinctions between virtues and skills; the difficulties in defining such words as *disposition* and *habit* as used in the traditional sense; the relationshp between natural and supernatural virtues; the relations of virtue, values, and concepts of the good, the unity or nonunity of the virtues, whether they are teachable or not, their relevance to health and medical care, and their relationship with duties, rights, and obligations.

MacIntyre, as we have said, extends the Aristotelian concept of virtue from internal qualities to practices, traditions of interpreting the good in specific communities; Hauerwas relates the virtues to the narrative of a particular people.[42] Some commentators are more critical, some more accepting, of the classical concepts. In the end the great majority say almost the same thing as ancient philosophers, but in more modern language. One is tempted to say of virtue, as it has been said of pornography, "I can't define it but I know it when I see it."

THE VIRTUOUS PERSON, THE VIRTUOUS PHYSICIAN

A set of common themes seems discernible in these many definitions. Virtue implies a character trait, an internal disposition haibtually to seek moral perfection, to live one's life in accord with the moral law, and to attain a balance between noble intention and just action. Perhaps Lewis has captured the idea best by likening the virtuous man to the good tennis player:

> What you mean by a good player is the man whose eye, muscles and nerves have been so trained by making innumerable good shots that they can be relied upon. . . . They have a certain tone or quality which is there even when he is not playing. . . . In the same way a man who perseveres in doing just actions gets in the end a certain quality of character. Now it is that quality rather than the particular actions that we mean when we talk of virtue.[43]

In almost any view the virtuous person is someone we can trust to act habitually in a good way—courageously, honestly, justly, wisely, and temperately. He or she is committed to *being* a good person and to the pursuit of perfection in private, professional, and communal life. The person is someone who will act well even when there is no one to applaud, simply because to act otherwise is a violation of what it is to be a good human being. No civilized society could endure without a significant number of citizens committed to this concept of virtue. Without such persons, no system of general ethics would succeed and no system of professional ethics could transcend the dangers of self-interest. That is why, even while rights, duties, and obligations may be emphasized, the concept of virtue has hovered so persistently over every system of ethics.

Is the virtuous physician simply the virtuous person practicing medicine? Are these virtues peculiar to medicine as a practice? Are certain of the individual virtues more applicable to medicine than elsewhere in human activities? Is virtue more important in some branches of medicine than others? How do professional skills differ from virtue? These are pertinent questions propaedeutic to the later question of the place of virtue in professional medical ethics.

We believe these questions are best answered by drawing on the notion of virtue and its relationship to the ends and purposes of human life. The virtuous physician, in this view, is defined in terms of the ends of medicine. To be sure, the physician, before anything else, must be a virtuous person. To be a virtuous physician, one must also be the kind of person we can confidently expect will be disposed to the right and good intrinsic to the practice professed. What are those dispositions?

To answer this question requires some exposition of what we mean by the good in medicine, or more specifically the good of the patient—for that is the end the patient and the physician ostensibly seek. Any theory of virtue must be linked with a theory of good because virtue is a disposition habitually to do the good. We must, therefore, know the nature of the good the virtuous person is disposed to do. As with the definition of virtue, we are caught here in another perennial philosophical question—what is the nature of The Good? Is The Good whatever we make it to be, or does it have validity independent of our desires or interest? Is The Good one or many? Is it reducible to riches, honors, pleasures, glory, happiness, or something else entirely?

We make no pretense about a discussion of a general theory of The Good. But any attempt to define the virtuous physician or a virtue-based ethic for medicine must offer some definition of the good of the patient. The patient's good is the end of medicine, that which shapes the particular virtues required for its attainment. That end is central to any notion of the virtues peculiar to medicine as a practice.

We have argued in chapter 4 that the architectonic principle of medicine is the good of the patient as expressed in a particular right and good healing action. This is the immediate good end of the clinical encounter. Health, healing, caring, and coping are all good ends dependent upon the more immediate end of a right and good decision. In this view the virtuous physician is one so habitually disposed to act in the patient's good by placing that good, in ordinary instances, above his own that he can reliably be expected to do so.

But we must face the fact that the patient's good is itself a compound notion. In chapters 3 and 4 we examined four components of the patient's good: (1) clinical or biomedical good; (2) the good as perceived by the patient; (3) the good of the patient as a human person; and (4) The Good, or ultimate good. Each of these components of patient good must be served.

Some would consider patient good, so far as the physician is concerned, as limited to what applied medical knowledge can achieve in *this* patient. In this view the virtues specific to medicine would be objectivity, scientific probity, and conscientiousness with regard to professional skill. One could perform the technical tasks of medicine per se, but without being a virtuous person. Would one then be a virtuous physician? One would have to answer yes if technical skill were all there is to medicine.

Some of the more expansionist models of medicine—such as Engel's bio-psychosocial model or that of the World Health Organization (total well-being)—would require compassion, empathy, advocacy, benevolence, and beneficence, that is, an expanded sense of the affective responses to patient need.[44] Some might argue that what is required, therefore, is not virtue but simply greater skill in the social and behavioral sciences applied to particular patients. In this view the physician's habitual dispositions might be incidental to his or her communication skills or empathy. One could achieve the ends of medicine without necessarily being a virtuous person in the generic sense.

It is important at this juncture to distinguish the virtues from technical or professional skills, as do MacIntyre and, more thoroughly, Von Wright. The latter defines a skill as "technical goodness" (excellence in some particular activity), while virtues are not tied to any one activity but are necessary for "the good of man."[45] The virtues are not "characterized" in terms of their results. In this view the technical skills of medicine are not virtues and could be practiced by a nonvirtuous person. Aristotle held *technē* (technical skills) to be one of the five intellectual virtues but not one of the moral virtues. It creates excellence but not moral worth.

The virtues enable the physician to act with regard to things that are good for man, when man is in the specific existential state of illness. They are dispositions always to seek the good intent inherent in healing. Within medicine the virtues do become, in MacIntyre's sense, acquired human qualities," the possession and exercise of which tends to enable us to achieve those goods which are internal to practices and the lack of which effectively prevents us from achieving any such goods."[46]

We come closer to the relationships of virtue to clinical actions if we look to the more immediate ends of medical encounters, to those moments of clinical truth when specific decisions and actions are chosen and carried out. The good the patient seeks is to be healed—to be restored to his or her prior, or a better, state of function, to be made "whole" again. If this is not possible, the patient expects to be helped, to be assisted in coping with the pain, disability, or dying that illness may entail. The immediate end of medicine is not simply a technically proficient performance but the use of that performance to attain a good end, the good of the patient—her medical or biomedical good to the extent possible, of course, but also the good as the patient perceives it, the good as a human person who can make a life plan, and the good as a person with a spiritual destiny, if this is her belief. It is the sensitive balancing of these sorts of patient good that the virtuous physician pursues to perfection.

To achieve the end of medicine thus conceived, to practice medicine virtuously, requires certain dispositions—conscientious attention to technical knowledge and skill, to be sure, but also compassion, a capacity to feel something of the patient's experience of illness and her perceptions of what is worthwhile; beneficence and benevolence, doing and wishing to do good for the patient; honesty, fidelity to promises; perhaps at times courage as well—the whole list of virtues spelled out by Aristotle: "justice, courage, temperance, magnanimity, liberality, placability, prudence, wisdom."[47] Not every one of these virtues is required in every decision. As we said, what we expect of the virtuous physician is that he or she will exhibit these virtues when they are required and that she will be so habitually disposed to do so that we can depend on it. She will place the good of the patient above her own and will seek that good unless its pursuit imposes an injustice upon her or her family, or requires a violation of her own conscience or professional standards. This balance between the patient's good and professional obligations forms the basis of the act of profession found in our last chapter.

While the virtues are necessary to attain the good internal to medicine as a practice, they exist independently of medicine. They are necessary for the practice of a good life, no matter in what activities that life may express itself. Certain of the virtues may become duties in the Stoic sense because of the nature of medicine as a practice. Medicine calls forth benevolence, beneficence, truth-telling, honesty, fidelity, and justice more than physical courage, for example. Yet even physical courage may be necessary when caring for the wounded on battlefields or in plagues, earthquakes, or other disasters. On a more ordinary scale, courage is necessary in treating contagious diseases, violent patients, or war casualties. Doing the right and good thing in medicine requires a more regular, intensive, and selective practice of the virtues than do many other callings.

A person can cultivate the technical skills of medicine for reasons other than the good of the patient—her own pride, profit, prestige, power. Such a physician can make technically right decisions and perform skillfully, but she could not be considered virtuous. She could not be depended upon to act against her own self-interest for the good of her patient.

In the virtuous physician, explicit fulfillment of rights and duties is an outward expression of an inner disposition to do the right and the good. One is virtuous not because one has conformed to the letter of the law or one's moral duties, but because that is what a good person does. One starts always with one's commitment to be a certain kind of person and then approaches clinical quandaries, conflicts of values, and patient interests as a good person ought.

Some branches of medicine would seem to demand a stricter and broader adherence to virtue than others. Generalists, for example, who deal with the more sensitive facets and nuances of a patient's history and humanity, must exercise the virtues more diligently than technique-oriented specialists. The narrower the specialty, the more easily the patient's good can be safeguarded by rules, regulations, rights, and duties; the broader the specialty, the more significant are the physician's character traits. No branch of medicine, however, can be practiced without some dedication to some of the virtues.

Unfortunately, physicians can compartmentalize their lives. Some practice medicine properly yet are guilty of vice in their lives. Others pay little attention to the character of their relationships with those to whom they owe special obligations. There are abundant examples of physicians who sincerely appear to seek the good of their patients and neglect obligations to their own family or friends. Some boast of being "married" to medicine and use this excuse to justify all sorts of failures in their other human relationships. We would not call such a person a virtuous physician. We could not be secure in, or trust, his disposition to act in a right and good way even in medicine. After all, one of the essential aspects of the virtues is balancing conflicting obligations judiciously. Further, a characteristic of virtue is its habituations, not seen in a compartmentalized sort of life.

As Socrates pointed out to Meno, one cannot really be virtuous piecemeal:

Why, did not I ask you to tell me the nature of virtue as a whole? And you are very far from telling me this; but declare every action to be virtue which is done with a part of virtue; as though you had told me and I must already know the whole of virtue, and this too when frittered away into little pieces. And therefore my dear Meno, I fear that I must begin again, and repeat the same question, what is virtue? For otherwise, I can only say that every action done with a part of virtue is virtue; what else is the meaning of saying that every action done with justice is virtue? Ought I not to ask the question over again; for can anyone who does not know virtue know a part of virtue?[48]

VIRTUES, RIGHTS, AND DUTIES IN MEDICAL ETHICS

Frankena has neatly summarized the distinctions among virtue-, rights-, and duty-based ethics as follows:

> In an ED [ethics of duty] then, the basic concept is that a certain kind of external act (or *doing*) to be done in certain circumstances; and that of a certain disposition being a virtue is a dependent one. In an EV [ethics of virtue] the basic concept is that a disposition or way of *being*—something one has, or is, not does—as a virtue, or as morally good; and that of an action's being virtuous or good or even right, is a dependent one.[49]

There are some logical difficulties with a virtue-based ethic that we must now note. For one thing, there must be some consensus on a definition of virtue. For another, there is a circularity in the assertion that virtue is what the good person habitually does, and that at the same time one becomes virtuous by doing good. Virtue and good are defined in terms of each other, and the definitions of both may vary among sincere people in actual practice when there is no other consensus, for example, regarding principles. A virtue-based ethics is difficult to defend as the sole basis for normative judgments, to say the least, in light of these weaknesses.

But note how this is a deficiency in rights- and duty-based ethics as well, which also must be linked to a theory of the good. In contemporary ethics, theories of virtue are rarely explicitly linked to theories of the right and good. Von Wright, commendably, is one of the few contemporary authorities who explicitly connects his theory of good with his theory of virtue.

By contrast, most professional ethical codes intermingle virtue and duty. The Hippocratic oath, for example, imposes certain duties such as protection of confidentiality, avoiding abortion, and not harming the patient. But the Hippocratic physician also pledges, "In purity and holiness, I will guard my life and my art." This is an exhortation to be a good person and a virtuous physician in order to serve patients in an ethically responsible way. Likewise, in one of the most humanistic statements in medical literature, the first-century writer Scribonius Largus made *humanitias* (compassion) an essential virtue. It thus becomes a role-specific duty. In claiming this, he was applying the Stoic doctrine of virtue to medicine.[50]

The 1980 version of the AMA Principles of Medical Ethics similarly intermingles duties, rights, and exhortations to virtues. It speaks of "standards of behavior," "essentials of honorable behavior," dealing "honestly" with patients and colleagues, and exposing colleagues "deficient in character." The Declaration of Geneva, which must meet the challenge of the widest array of value systems, nonetheless calls for practice "with conscience and dignity" in keeping with "the honor and noble traditions of the profession."[51] Though their first allegiance must be to the Communist ethos, even Soviet physicians are urged to preserve "the high title of physician," "to keep and develop the beneficial traditions of medicine," and to "dedicate" all their "knowledge and strength to the care of the sick." These virtues are not unlike the June 1983 American Board of

Internal Medicine's policy requiring "high standards of humanistic behavior in the professional lives of every certifiable candidate."[52]

Those who are cynical of any protestation of virtue on the part of physicians will interpret these excerpts as the last remnants of a dying tradition of altruistic benevolence. But, at the very least, they attest to the recognition that the good of the patient cannot be fully protected by rights and duties alone. Some degree of supererogation is built into the nature of the relationship between those who are ill and those who profess to help them.

This, too, may be why many graduating classes, still idealistic about their calling, choose the prayer of Maimonides (not by Maimonides at all) over the more deontological oath of Hippocrates. In that "prayer" the physician asks, "May neither avarice nor miserliness, nor thirst for glory or for a great reputation engage my mind; for the enemies of truth and philanthropy may easily deceive me and make me forgetful of my lofty aim of doing good to thy children." This is an unequivocal call to virtue, and it is hard to imagine even the most cynical graduate failing to comprehend its message.

All professional medical codes, then, are built on a three-tiered system of obligations related to the special roles of physicians in society. In ascending order of ethical sensitivity they are observance of the laws of the land, observance of rights and fulfillment of duties, and, finally, the practice of virtue.

At the next level is the ethics of rights and duties that spells out obligations beyond those defined by law. Here benevolence and beneficence take on more than their legal meanings. The ideal of service, of responsiveness to the special needs of those who are ill, some degree of compassion, kindliness, promise-keeping, truth-telling and nonmaleficence, and specific obligations such as confidentiality and autonomy are included. How these principles are applied, and conflicts among them resolved in the patient's best interests, are subjects of widely varying interpretations. How sensitively these issues are confronted depends more on the physician's character than on his or her capability at ethical discourse or moral casuistry.

Virtue-based ethics goes beyond these first two levels. We expect the virtuous person to do the right and the good even at the expense of personal sacrifice and legitimate self-interest. Virtue ethics expands the notions of benevolence, beneficence, conscientiousness, compassion, and fidelity well beyond what strict duty might require. It makes some degree of supererogation mandatory because it calls for standards of ethical performance that exceed those prevalent in the rest of society.[53] We developed this point by contrasting our view with Goldman's in the last chapter.

At each of these three levels, there are certain dangers from overzealous or misguided observance. Legalistic ethical systems tend toward a justification of minimalist ethics, a narrow definition of benevolence or beneficence, and a contract-minded physician-patient relationship. Rights- and duty-based ethics may be distorted by overly strict rule worship and adherence to the letter of ethical principles without the modulations and nuances the spirit of those principles implies. A virtue-based ethics, being the least specific, can more easily lapse into self-righteous paternalism or an unwelcome overinvolvement in the personal life of the patient. Misapplication of any moral system, even with good intent, converts benevolence into maleficence. The virtuous person might be expected to be more sensitive to these aberrations, because of the requirement of balance, than someone whose ethics is more deontologically or legally flavored.

The more we yearn for ethical sensitivity, the less we lean on rights, duties, rules, and principles and the more on the character traits of the moral agent. Paradoxically, without rules, rights, and duties specifically spelled out, we cannot predict what form a particular person's expression of virtue will take. In a pluralistic society, as we argued in the previous chapter, principles and professional standards ought to assure a dependable minimum level of moral conduct. But that minimal level is insufficient in the complex, often unpredictable circumstances of decision making, where technical and value desiderata intersect so inextricably.

The virtuous physician does not act from unreasoned, uncritical intuitions about what feels good. His or her disposition stems, instead, from order in accord with the "right reason" that both Aristotle and Aquinas considered essential to virtue. Medicine is itself ultimately an exercise of practical wisdom—a right way of acting in difficult and uncertain circumstances for a specific end, that is, the good of a particular person who is ill. It is when the choice of a right and good action becomes most difficult, when the temptations to self-interest are most insistent, when unexpected nuances of good and evil arise, and when no one is looking that the differences between an ethics based in virtue and an ethics based in law and/or duty can most clearly be distinguished.

Virtue-based professional ethics distinguishes itself, therefore, less by the avoidance of overtly immoral practices than by the avoidance of practices at the margin of moral respectability. Physicians are confronted, in today's morally relaxed climate, with an increasing number of new practices that pit altruism against self-interest. Most are not illegal or, strictly speaking, immoral in a rights- or duty-based ethic. But they are not consistent with the higher levels of moral sensitivity that a virtue-based ethics demands. These practices can be grouped into four categories: (1) making a profit from the illness of others, (2) narrowing the concept of service for personal convenience, (3) taking a proprietary attitude with respect to medical knowledge, and (4) placing loyalty to the profession above loyalty to patients.

Under the first heading we might include such things as investment in and ownership of for-profit hospitals, hospital chains, nursing homes, and dialysis units; tie-in arrangements with radiological or laboratory services; escalation of fees for repetitive, high-volume procedures, and lax indications for the use of such procedures, especially when third-party payers allow such charges.

The second type of morally questionable practice might include the ever-decreasing availability and accessibility of physicians; the diffusion of individual patient responsibility in group practices so that the patient never knows whom he will see or who is on call; the itinerant emergency room physician who works two days and skis three, with little commitment to hospital or community; and the growing overindulgence by physicians in vacations, recreation, and "self-development."

The third category might include such practices as "selling one's services" for whatever the market will bear; providing what the market demands and not necessarily what the community needs; patenting new procedures or keeping them secret from potential competitor-colleagues; looking at the investment of time, effort, and capital in a medical education as justification for "making it back"; and for forgetting that medical knowledge is drawn from the cumulative experience of a multitude of patients, clinicians, and investigators.

Under the last category might be included referrals on the basis of friendship and reciprocity rather than skill; resisting consultations and second opinions as affronts to one's competence; placing the interests of the referring physician above those of one's patients; and looking the other way in the face of incompetence or even dishonesty in one's professional colleagues.

These and many other practices are defended and even encouraged by sincere physicians in today's era of competition. Some can be quite properly rationalized in a deontological ethics, but it would be impossible to envision a physician committed to the virtues who would assent to these practices. A virtue-based ethics simply does not fluctuate with what the dominant social mores will tolerate. It must interpret benevolence, beneficence, and responsibility in a way that reduces self-interest and enhances altruism. This is the only convincing answer the profession can give to the growing perception that medicine is nothing more than a business and should be regulated as such.

A virtue-based ethics is inherently elitist, in the best sense, because its adherents demand more of themselves than does the prevailing morality. It calls forth that extra measure of dedication that has made the best physicians in every era exemplars of what the human spirit can achieve. No matter to what depths a society may fall, virtuous persons will always be the beacons that light the way back to moral sensitivity; virtuous physicians ought to be the beacons that show the way back to moral credibility for the whole profession.

We believe that Jonsen rightly diagnoses the central paradox in medicine as the tension between self-interest and altruism.[54] No amount of deft juggling of rights, duties, or principles will suffice to resolve that tension. We are all too good at rationalizing what we want to do so that personal gain can be converted from vice to virtue. Only a character formed by the virtues can detect such intellectual hypocrisy.

To be sure, the twin themes of self-interest and altruism have been inextricably joined in the history of medicine. There have always been physicians who reject the virtues or, more often, claim them falsely. But there have also been physicians, more often than the critics of medicine would allow, who have been truly virtuous. They have been, and remain, the leaven of the profession and the hope of all who are ill. They form the seawall that will not be eroded even by the powerful forces of commercialization, bureaucratization, and mechanization inevitable in modern medicine.

We cannot, need not, and, indeed, must not wait for a medical analogue of MacIntyre's "new Saint Benedict" to show us the way. There is no new concept of virtue waiting to be discovered that is peculiarly suited to the dilemmas of our own dark age. We must recapture the courage to speak of character, virtue, and perfection in living a good life. We must encourage those who are willing to dedicate themselves to a higher standard of self-effacement, as we shall explore in our penultimate chapter.

We need the courage, too, to accept the obvious split in the profession between those who see and feel the altruistic imperatives in medicine and those who do not. Those who at heart believe that the pursuit of private self-interest serves the public good are very different from those who believe in restraining self-interest. We forget that physicians since the beginnings of the profession have subscribed to different values and virtues. We need only recall that the Hippocratic oath was taken by physicians of the Pythagorean school at the time when most Greek physicians followed essentially a craft ethic.[55] A perusal of the Hippocratic corpus itself, which intersperses ethics and etiquette, will show how differently its treatises deal with fees, the care of incurable patients, and the business aspects of the craft.

The illusion that all physicians share a common devotion to a high-flown set of ethical principles has done damage to medicine by raising expectations some members of the profession cannot or will not fulfill. Today we must be more forthright about the differences in value commitment among physicians. Professional codes must be more explicit about the relationships between duties, rights, and virtues. Such explicitness encourages a more honest relationship between physicians and patients, and removes the hypocrisy of verbal assent to a general code to which an individual physician may not really subscribe. Explicitness enables patients to choose among physicians on the basis of their ethical commitments, as well as their reputations for technical expertise.

Conceptual clarity will not assure virtuous behavior. Indeed, virtues are usually distorted if they are the subject of too conscious a design. But conceptual clarity will distinguish between motives and provide criteria for judging the moral commitment one can expect from the profession and its individual members. It can also inspire those whose virtuous inclinations need reinforcement in the current climate of commercialization of the healing relationship.

To this end the current resurgence of interest in virtue-based ethics is altogether salubrious. Linked to a theory of patient good and a theory of rights and duties, it can provide the needed groundwork for a reconstruction of professional medical ethics as that work matures. Perhaps even more progress can be made if we take Shakespeare's advice in Hamlet: "Assume the virtue if you have it not. . . . For use almost can change the stamp of nature."

III

THE CONSEQUENCES
OF BENEFICENCE

10

The Common Devotion:
A Reconstruction of Medical Ethics

Hope remains only in the most difficult task of all: *to reconsider everything from the ground up,* so as to shape a living
society in a dying society.
A. Camus, *Neither Victims Nor Executioners*

Like his colleague William Osler, Harvey Cushing was one of those extraordinary men who graced our profession as much by his dedication to humane learning as by his contributions to scientific medicine. Like Osler, too, he had a special dedication to the moral imperatives that bind all who profess to care for the
sick. That dedication is the one ligature that holds all physicians together, no
matter in what age, speciality, or cultural era they practice. That dedication, too,
is what Cushing called our "common devotion" in his commencement address
at the Jefferson Medical College in June 1926.[1]

It is significant that Cushing entitled that address *Consecratio Medici* (the
doctor's consecration), which he defined as a commitment to a "higher" standard of self-effacement."[2] Cushing chose this theme because he felt that certain
trends in his day threatened the physician's fealty to the good of his patients. He
deplored the debasement of clinical skills, the overemphasis on research, and
the pursuit of personal gain that he perceived in his colleagues. The list sounds
surprisingly up-to-date. To counter these trends Cushing exhorted the graduating class to put the patient's good above self-interest—to rededicate themselves
to what must be their "common devotion."

Cushing's call to a common devotion by his generation is his legacy. That
legacy calls upon every generation of physicians to establish and refurbish its
own moral credentials. It is our obligation to examine the requirements of moral
credibility for our profession in the face of the dilemmas, catastrophes, and
opportunities of our day.

In his time Cushing could exhort his colleagues simply to reaffirm a heritage

127

of common values shared more or less universally by his contemporaries. He called on them to reaffirm the Hippocratic oath, to emulate the nobler physicians of literature and history, and to return to medicine "something of its quondam religious significance."[3]

Our times are more complex and divisive than Cushing's. The Hippocratic ethic is no longer the universally accepted guide it was then;[4] the doctors in our novels are picaresque heroes, to be pitied more than emulated; history in our self-centered age is ignored or scorned, and religion has lost much of its influence in practical affairs. While many of the principles of our traditional medical ethos are still valid, they must be reexamined, expanded, and refined, as we have done in the previous chapters. Here we examine the implications of a lack of consensus about our medical task.

THE WEAKENED EDIFICE OF MEDICAL ETHICS

The foundations of a common devotion, the moral cement of shared values that Cushing could presume, have been greatly weakened since his time. Many of the dicta of the Hippocratic oath are being questioned, while many of our most crucial ethical questions are simply not addressed.[5,6] In addition, physicians, families, and patients reflect the moral relativism, and even amoralism, of our time. We are acrimoniously divided on the most fundamental issues of human life, such as abortion, euthansia, prolonging life or letting patients die, and the use of reproductive technologies. We disagree on the most common questions technology places before us: Who shall live? Who shall die? Who shall decide? How? These questions scarcely arose in Cushing's time.

Two recent examples will suffice to illustrate the disarray of contemporary medical ethics: treatment of the dying patient and treatment of seriously malformed infants.

The first is exemplified by a series of articles entitled "As They Lay Dying" in the Washington Post the week of April 17, 1983.[7] Here we see documented the torment of conscientious physicians making the most urgent moral choices about living and dying. Physician after physician, who worked in emergency rooms, intensive care units, coronary care units, nursing homes, and hospices gave eloquent testimony to the frustrations of trying to serve the conflicting demands of technological possibility, fiscal constraint, and the discordant values of patients, families, and the law. Even more revealing was the clear absence of any moral consensus, or of a clear and orderly way to approach the most common clinical dilemmas.

It is ironic that at the very moment in history that medicine's technological capabilities are in such ascendancy, cost-cutting measures seem to freeze our abilities to treat patients with all the means at our disposal. In an article about new laser technologies that make neurosurgery a much more gentle art than it was in the past, Cerullo argues that neurosurgeons should superspecialize. He prefers to operate on tumors only with lasers. In the future, he thinks, physicians will sit at computer consoles, "pushing buttons to direct lasers to silently pass through the skull and melt away the tumor." And yet prepaid health plans such as health maintenance organizations do not even want to pay for a computerized axial tomography (CAT) scan since, if the scan is negative, they lose money. Cerullo cites the case of a woman complaining of double vision who, after being refused twice by the HMO, paid for her own CAT scan. The results showed a tumor pressing on the optic nerve. Much of her vision loss was, by then, irreversible. Cerullo muses that patients in an HMO will have little chance to see the superspecialists of the future.[8]

The second example is the dilemma posed in two cases of infants with Down's syndrome and easily correctable surgical malformations of the gastrointestinal tract. In the much-publicized *Baby Doe* case, the highest court in Indiana upheld the demand on the parents to withhold surgery while medical opinion was divided. In a parallel case in Leicester, England, the court ordered surgery over the objections of the family and the attending surgeon.

We must assume that the parties in these two cases were well intentioned. Certainly, in each case, they felt they were sincerely acting in the best interests of the infant. On one side the intent was to spare it a burdensome life of "low" quality; on the other, to afford it a chance at life of some quality not precisely predictable. On our most forcefully cited justification for moral choice—the patient's good—the courts, the physicians, and the patients' surrogates differed drastically.

The same contradictions occur in treating comatose and terminal patients, in decisions to treat or withhold treatment from the elderly, or to respect a living will. Indeed, in almost every important clinical decision, there can be wide discrepancies in views of what is right and good. There are radical differences in the sources of medical morality—in the philosophical and theological foundations on which physicians and others base their moral choices. It is obvious that the intention to do the "right thing" does not guarantee that an act will be good unless we accept an absolute moral relativism and a situational ethics that leads to moral anarchy. By using different moral assumptions, well-intentioned persons can arrive at differing conclusions.

Not only have our common belief systems been eroded, but so, even, has the idea of ethics as a defensible enterprise. During the Enlightenment, for example, reasonableness and balance were the norm for scientific humanism. People gained control of the political enterprise and trusted not only in the institutions they created and controlled but also in one another. Today the opposite seems to be the case. People no longer trust science and technology, their institutions, or one another. They do not share a common cultural moral perspective. In this atmosphere it is difficult to propose universal standards of good and ill, or to critique hierarchies of values from any standard perspective.[9]

Where do physicians, as morally accountable individuals and members of a morally accountable profession, turn for help? There has been no dearth of debate in these issues outside professional precincts. Ethicists have produced an enormous literature analyzing such concepts as autonomy, paternalism, killing and letting die, and the application of most of the principles of general ethics to medicine. The courts have intervened when moral disagreements impeded decisions or threatened the legal rights of the participants.[10] Ethics committees have been established to advise and to negotiate differences. A president's commission has made voluminous recommendations on such topics as defining death, making health decisions, protecting human subjects, and foregoing life-sustaining treatments.[11] The FTC has taken the radical step of declaring professional codes to be nothing more than self-serving devices in restraint of trade.

Nevertheless, the ethicists' distinctions must eventually be tested in the clinical arena. Courts do not establish morality; neither committees, nor even the pronouncements of prestigious presidential commissions or the FTC, absolve from personal moral accountability. The painful fact remains that moral considerations override all others and that each member of the profession is responsible for his or her own moral credibility as well as that of the profession.

This fact must be faced today without the traditional security of a noble, unfailing, universally respected code of ethics. The recent revisions of the AMA code, the Hippocratic oath, and the many codes derived from it continue to be useful. But they are inadequate for the most crucial ethical questions of our day: How do we assure that moral choices among persons whose values and ethical systems may vary widely can be made in a morally defensible way? How do we preserve our personal moral accountability in a pluralistic society and still assure our patients that we will respect their moral potentialities? Without deprecating existing codes, we must recognize that they have lost some of their force because they presuppose a homogeneity of philosophical and even theological values that no longer exists. With so many differences at so many fundamental levels, is medical ethics doomed to frustrating atomization?

TOWARD A RECONSTRUCTION OF MEDICAL ETHICS

We believe medical ethics can be solidly reconstructed. That reconstruction must be from the ground up—that is, it must be based in the one irreducible foundation of all clinical medicine, the relationship between one who seeks health and one who professes to help and heal.[12] There are three requirements for redesigning the architecture of medical ethics consistent with today's dilemmas:

1. It must be modular in construction.
2. It must incorporate a clear notion of what constitutes the good of the patients.
3. It must renovate and refurbish the traditional ideal of a profession.

The remainder of this chapter is devoted to an elaboration of these three requirements.

The Modular Approach to Medical Morality

We have long been accustomed to thinking of medical ethics in terms of a uniform code or as a single set of self-contained, self-justifying principles. The erosion of a common philosophical and theological belief system makes this concept no longer tenable. Instead, a complete medical ethics might consist of four components, closely linked and interdependent, yet separable in actual ethical discourse and moral choice.

The first module consists of the positions we take on the specific ethical issues of the day, such as euthanasia, abortion, terminating treatment, living wills, artificial insemination—any of the multitude of new questions put before us by our technological capability. Much of the strife of ethical discourse and decision arises from opposing positions on these issues. Most people simply assert their positions as right and good and reject any argument that exposes the sources of their opinions.

The second module contains the philosophical sources upon which the positions in the first module are based. These are encompassed by three large categories: (1) the theory of ethics to which we subscribe—deontological, utilitarian, contractarian, consequentialist, or teleological; (2) the construal we place on the fundamental ethical principles of truth-telling, promise-keeping, beneficence, nonmaleficence, justice, and the like; and (3) the concept we hold of the nature, destiny, and worth of human existence.

The third module comprises our theological and religious beliefs: what we think about God, our duties to him, and the ultimate destiny and meaning of human existence. The positions taken on these questions by believers and nonbelievers alike seriously affect their moral choices.

The fourth module is less well developed than the other three. Unlike them, it is not substantive in content but deals with the ethics of the process of interpersonal moral decision making. It comprises our position on such things as patient participation, strong and weak paternalism, libertarianism, protecting the autonomy and moral agency of the patient, telling the truth, manipulating consent, and handling conflicts between the interacting parties—physicians, members of other health professions, patients, and patients' families. This module should aim at assuring a morally defensible transaction between persons who may differ widely on the substantive ethical issues and who yet must enter a medical transaction with each other. This is the ethics of a moral relationship between physicians and patients irrespective of what their positions may be on specific medical-moral questions.

Out of the interaction between these four modules of medical ethics we arrive at what we think is right and good in a particular clinical situation. A complete and mature medical morality requires us to be clear about our positions in each module. Only then can we understand the basis for our own actions, and where, and at what level, we disagree or agree with patients and others involved in clinical decisions.

It is unlikely that we will ever again enjoy wide agreement on the philosophical or theological sources of our medical morality. It is therefore unlikely that we can achieve general agreement on specific clinical moral decisions. If any common principles are possible, they will probably be deducible only in the fourth component—in a procedural ethics that respects the obligations of each person to be faithful to his or her own belief systems.

Development of this fourth module is presently our most urgent need in medical ethics in a democratic society. The Hippocratic corpus says very little about the process of making decisions. If anything, it is strongly paternalistic and even warns against sharing information with the patient. The most recent revision of the AMA code is silent on this subject, though it is treated under the heading of informed consent in the Opinions of the Judicial Council.[13] On the whole, the most vexed questions about who decides, and how, are still left largely to individual interpretation.

This deficiency is no longer acceptable. Patients and their families want to know how physicians will make decisions, who will have the final say, and how physicians will handle potential conflict. They will also increasingly want to know our position on the major medical-moral questions. This is becoming a central issue on the agenda of medical ethics in the immediate future.

Ethics of the Process of Moral Choice in Clinical Ethics

The possibilities of conflict between various modules of medical ethics and the good of the patient underscore the need for a careful definition of which good we mean when we defend a specific clinical decision. It also implies some ranking of these various senses of patient good. We have discussed this matter at length in chapter 6, and only summarize it here.

Ultimate good is the highest sense of the patient's good. Recall that this sense was the value to which an individual appealed as a first and last resort. For many persons this is God. For others it is the driving force of their life, their ultimate concern.

The second highest sense of patient good for a competent patient is that which preserves his or her capacity to act in a fully human way, that is, to express and act on her own perception of her own good. That good is owed every patient simply because she is human. If the patient is not competent, her surrogate or proxy is expected to ascertain what choice the patient would have made. The patient's freedom to choose is limited only when it poses some direct, immediate, and discernible harm to another person, or if fulfilling the patient's perception of good would violate the physician's conscience. The physician, as well as the patient, is a moral agent and, as such, cannot be expected to cooperate in what he or she considers to be wrong.

The patient's conception of her own good ranks right behind her good as a human person. It takes precedence over biomedical good or medical indications. To force medical good on the patient, or to accomplish it by deception or manipulation for the "patient's good," is to violate the patient's good as a human being and as the agent of her own moral choices.

Biomedical good and medical indications are, therefore, lowest in the hierarchy of senses in which we can interpret the good of the patient. Beneficial as they might be, they do not justify violation of the higher good of the patient as a human being to express her own choices and to determine the specific nature of what is in her best interests.

An ethics of the process of clinical moral choices, therefore, obligates the physician to respect the several dimensions of the good of the patient and to keep them distinct and in proper order when they are in conflict. Some of these obligations are described below.

Refurbishing the Traditional Idea of the Profession

In all decisions the physician has the responsibility for an objective assessment of biomedical good, that is, how the proposed treatment will change the short- and long-term prognosis and history of the disease. That assessment must be objective, scientifically sound, and free of quality-of-life judgments if these place external value on the life of another person. In this way the patient (or his surrogate) is enabled to determine accurately what choices she is being asked to make.

The assessment of the good to be achieved by a medical intervention should be presented as sensitively and clearly as possible. It must be fitted to the patient's educational, cultural, linguistic, and ethnic background. The physician has an obligation to assist the patient to make as cogent a choice as possible— and to do so without coercion or deception.

After they have been properly and sensitively informed, some patients may ask the physician to make the decision for them. The physician then has a mandate to do so. Having a mandate is very different from taking a strongly paternalistic role from the outset.

With an incompetent or never-competent patient, the physician should accord the same freedom of choice to the surrogates. She then has the additionally difficult obligations to be sure that the surrogate is competent to make the decision and that, in addition, the surrogate is acting in the best interests of the patient.

The whole process is greatly complicated in the case of infants. Here the family's wishes and their quality-of-life determinants may color the decision. But the physician's concern must be for the infant, for the infant, not the family, is the patient. In the never-competent patient there is no way to ascertain what the patient would see as her interests. Therefore, medical good, the probability of improving the patient's functioning or comfort, assumes a more dominant place than in the case of the competent or once-competent patient.

When serious moral disagreements between physicians or surrogates occur, especially in the case of infants, recourse should be had to some judicious, uninvolved deliberative group—a consultant, an ethics committee, a court-appointed guardian. If all this fails, court intervention may be necessary. But this is not the way to determine what is morally right; it is only a lesser way of determining which decision is to be made, and to be sure that some decision is made that at least protects legal rights.

The best clinical decisions are those in which medical good, the patient's interests, and the freedom to choose are congruent—and in many cases they are. Most often, the differences can be negotiated if they are approached with trust and sensitivity, and without deception. The quality of the relationship between patients, families, and medical attendants, rather than rules of procedure or moral algorithms, will often be the deciding factor.

Unfortunately, the trusting relationship required for so momentous a decision as, let us say, a no-code order is becoming ever more difficult in contemporary medical care. Team care, multiple consultations, rotations of house staff, institutionalization, stress at the moment of decision—all complicate the relationship. In public and teaching hospitals, often there is no sustained relationship with the patient, no one who can serve as a personal physician in the delicate process of making moral choices. This is an intolerable impediment to ethical patient care in the complicated nexus of today's clinical decisions.

An ethics of moral decision making must also include respect for the moral agencies and moral accountability of all health professionals interacting in the clinical decision. The physician may have technical and even legal authority to perform certain acts, as may the nurse, social worker, and others. But because no one has moral authority over another, all members of the medical and health care teams are morally accountable first to themselves and then to their patients. Each promises to help and to act in the patient's best interests.

There will be times when orders cannot be followed because the moral principles of some team members would be violated. At other times, if some serious transgression of obligations to patients occurs, "whistle blowing," with all its painful consequences, may be necessary. Physicians need far more awareness and sensitivity to the potentialities for moral conflicts with the other health professions and must learn to deal with these conflicts in a way that respects the moral agencies of their colleagues.

CONCLUSION

Our moral choices are more difficult, more subtle, and more controversial than those of Cushing's time. We must make them without the heritage of shared values that could unify the medical ethics of his era. Our task is not to abandon hope in medical ethics, but to undertake what Camus called "the most difficult task of all: to reconsider everything from the ground up, so as to shape a living society inside a dying society."[14] That task is not the demolition of the edifice of medical morality, but its reconstruction along three lines we have delineated: (1) replacement of a monolithic with a modular structure for medical ethics, with special emphasis on the ethics of making moral choices in clinical decisions; (2) clarification of what we mean when we speak of the good of the patient, and setting some priority among the several senses in which that term may be taken; and (3) refurbishing the ideal of a profession as a true "consecration," in Cushing's phrase.

In this regard Olser, like Cushing, left a moral challenge as his legacy. In his last address on the occasion of his installation as president of the British Classical Association, he ended with a call to *philanthropia* and *philotechnia* (love of humanity and love of art).[15] Osler took his words from the legacy of another great physician, Hippocrates.

Will we, in our generation, be faithful to the legacy of these great physicians who saw so clearly that medicine is at heart a moral enterprise? Are we equal to the challenge of Cushing's *Consecratio Medici?* Our final chapter will present our suggestion for a straightforward act of profession based on this consecration, which also summarizes our work on beneficence in medicine.

11

Making Decisions Under Uncertainty

> The true art of thinking justly, and with precision;—the
> object most deserving the attention of man; the most solid
> fruit of science.
>
> Claude Buffier, *Traité des Premières Véritez,*
> *et de la Source de nos Jugemens.*

We have discussed the virtuous, or good, physician and the virtuous, or good, patient. When they meet each other, at the actual moment of clinical decision making, their values and beliefs must of necessity intersect. As virtuous persons, each will be desirous of doing what is right and good, and each will act in a morally responsible way.

How can this critical intersection of values be so conducted as to respect the moral integrity of the interacting parties? What constitutes a morally defensible decision-making process that will at the same time be analytically sound and technically competent?

In recent years much attention has been directed at making explicit the traditionally implicit process of clinical decisions. Can the principle of beneficence, which we have expounded in this book, be sustained in decision-making models of medicine?

In this chapter we will develop the thesis that decision-analysis theory must take into account the values of the patient in order to be a valid logic of the clinical relationship. We choose this particular theory of medical decision making because it appears to us to neglect the role of the patient in arriving at its conclusions, though it need not do so. Perhaps the reason why this has historically been the case is that the model has been applied to difficult clinical decisions involving two apparently equal outcomes in terms of "utilities" for the patient. We will therefore discuss the basic outline of decision-analysis methodology.

Patients make decisions. They do so about their health treatment plans in the context of the doctor-patient relation. From the time of Hippocrates to the present, doctors have argued that this relationship requires them to act in the best interest of their patients, even if that would mean sometimes violating a moral rule such as truth-telling.[1] Thus Henderson, in an oft-quoted passage, admonishes, "Try at all times to act upon the patient so as to modify his sentiments to his own advantage."[2] The reason for this admonition is that Henderson, like thousands of other physicians before and after him, holds that patients place a kind of faith in their doctors that requires the latter to act out of beneficence. This activity is so strongly expressed that doctors themselves are sometimes described as therapeutic agents.[3]

Since Henderson's time, though, major changes have taken place in medicine and in society itself. These changes have led to an emphasis on patient autonomy rather than on faith in the physician. The factors that have fostered a commitment to autonomy are the misuse of medicine for political aims; the rise of patient rights movements; better patient education; the depersonalization, institutionalization, and specialization of medicine; intense competitiveness in medical school; the rise of the medical-industrial complex; and the emergence of team health care.

The result has been a clash between traditional paternalism and the new emphasis on patient autonomy. Our thesis is that despite all of these changes, beneficence remains the primary principle that should ground the ethics of medicine. Our thesis is supported by three arguments corresponding to the three sections of this chapter: First, we will show how decision-analysis theory requires beneficence in its calculations of utilities and in its assessment of these utilities with patients. Second, we will analyze the special character of decisions that must be made by patients who face death. Third, we will argue that beneficence is essential in decision making with patients of diminished or compromised competence. Our argument examines the stages of increasing uncertainty about patient competence and outcomes. Finally, we will offer a critique of substituted judgment and the reasonable persons standard from the viewpoint of beneficence.

DECISION ANALYSIS

Decision analysis spells out in detail the steps involved in making a complex decision. Three types of decisions may occur in medicine: The first is decision under certainty, that is, when the choice directly determines outcomes; the second is decision under risk, when possible outcomes are known but their probability is uncertain; the third is decision under uncertainty, when we cannot or do not know the outcomes.[4-8]

In each type of decision, the consequences may be judged good (benefit), bad (hazards), or some mixture of good and bad. When a consequence of a decision has both good and bad components, we call that consequence a *utility*. In each of the three types of decision making, beneficence plays a predominant role. Let us look at each in more detail.

When decisions are made under certainty, the value of that outcome for the patient is determined, usually by the patient himself. We have written of such decisions as "making right and good" decisions "with" and "for" patients. By right we meant a medically correct decision made on the basis of medical indications and state-of-the-art interventions; by good we meant an ethically sound decision. Here, ethical probability is rooted in such concerns as the freedom of the patient, respect for the person, and the value of the expected consequence of the treatment for the patient. Thus, if a patient is concerned about hypertension and its consequences, and the physician finds that a salt-poor diet is indicated, the decision to begin such a diet would be a value decision. It would fulfill medical and moral requirements of the good. The diagnosis, recommendation, and jointly made decision would rest on the notion of benefit to the patient.

A more difficult decision, however, might be a recommendation to amputate fingers and toes currently causing intolerable pain to a patient suffering from rheumatoid arthritis. The outcome is certain. After a period of intense pain, the incisions will heal and the arthritic patient will be free of useless and painful joints. Here, by contrast, the "benefit" to the patient would be mixed. The patient would no longer be able to perform certain daily tasks, and some residual pain would continue in amputated limbs at the site of the amputation. Decision analysis would attempt to calculate mathematically the utilities of amputation versus other drastic measures of pain control. At this point, also, numbers cannot adequately express the complex of values involved in such a case. The patient's own value system is required to calculate (if we may use that word) utilities and make recommendations.

Evidence exists that patients do want physicians to be sources of information and to decide on their behalf, but they also want to have an input into the decision process. This evidence supports a theory of beneficence rather than autonomy. In the decision-making process, while pressing for more information, patients may not want to actually make the decision but rather to urge the physician to employ more effort in diagnosing and managing the problem. Vertinsky, Thompson, and Uyeno found, for example, that all two hundred randomly sampled patients in their study rated direct participation or patient decision as unimportant in the doctor-patient relation, yet all indicated a desire to maintain some measure of participation.[9] The authors of this study conclude that it supports the Szasz-Hollender "guidance-cooperation" model of the clinical relation.[10] If this is the case, then the physicians' "guidance" must be in the direction of what would benefit the patient. It appears that patients want to maintain their autonomy within the broader context of a relation of need, trust, and guidance. Bergsma found something similar in general practice, leading him to formulate a theory of shared autonomy.[11]

With decisions made under risk, it is our contention that the greater the uncertainty about which choice to make, the greater the need for beneficence. We base this contention on the following evidence: First, it is clear that people cannot process too much information at one time. At a certain point, overload is reached, expecially if important values are at stake.[12-14] At this point they need help in sorting out their own values in order to make a satisfactory decision.

This "help" must be sensitive at all times to the patient's values and not skewed in favor of the physician's values. Second, decision analysis can provide such help by carefully analyzing the risks and benefits and, from these calculations, arriving at a decision.[15] The reduction of values and utilities to numbers is made on the grounds that all actions, even those based on clinical hunches, involve assumptions about success, that is, probabilities. Decision analysis therefore compels the physician to distinguish medical facts (probability estimates) from patient attitudes about outcomes (utility functions). It is not clear, however, that mathematical calculations actually lead to beneficent decisions. Let us look at two examples, both provided by Pauker and Kassirer.[16]

In the first example, decision analysis is used to clarify a decision about the use of a diagnostic test with marginal benefit. A calculus of risks and benefits is used to assign quantitative weight to the value desiderata involved in the decision. These weights are arrived at statistically and, of course, may or may not apply to the individual patient under consideration. The "benefits" are based in avoiding complications, for example, using corticosteroids to treat malignant hypertension versus creating vasculitis.

Such an analysis seems overly mathematical and insensitive to the patient's values. This impression is borne out in another of Pauker and Kassirer's articles. In a case involving an elderly woman with suspected pulmonary emboli, they weigh the benefits and risks of pulmonary arteriography and long-term anticoagulant therapy. They claim that a "simple calculation" will eventuate in the "optimal choice" without taking into consideration the patient's values: "Because neither the patient nor her family were considered capable of comprehending the issues involved, the value judgments regarding both morbidity and mortality were made without their input."[17] One might argue that beneficence is the basis for the authors' decision, but we would argue instead that, unless patient and family were all incompetent, their values should have been a part of the calculus. The fact that such values cannot conveniently be mathematicized is not a moral warrant for ignoring them.[18,19]

Overmathematicization can be the nemesis of decision analysis, but it need not be. Weinstein and coworkers point out that input values are uncertain, and that the same raw data on Reye's syndrome led to two different conclusions in decision-analysis studies. Yet, as they point out, the purpose of decision analysis is not to establish scientific truth but to help make difficult decisions.[20] Brett argues that decision analysis based on mathematics alone will produce results heavily skewed toward intervention. One treatment may be better than another by minute differences. Yet the theory requires one to act in favor of the better strategy, "no matter how minute." Brett proposes that, in weighing means and ends, physicians must examine their own values about therapy and clinical results, and must encourage patients to do the same. In that way the principle of doing no harm, a subset of beneficence, can be protected. Brett recognized that patients under the duress of illness may not be able to make subtle value judgments and may ask their physicians to make the decision. He concludes that the concrete reality of the medical event is interaction with individuals, not manipulation of statistics.[21]

The importance of including and acting on patient value judgments is underscored by several other shortcomings of decision analysis. For example, to a patient who must choose between laryngectomy and radiotherapy for cancer of the larynx, the former may appear more desirable because it has a higher five-year survival rate (60 percent compared with 40 percent for radiotherapy). But a five-year survival statistic may not reflect quality of life or may not accurately reflect actual survival from the disease (for example, deaths from the surgery or radiotherapy itself may be included). One study of lung cancer survival reports: "This measure [five-year survival] implies that any death occurring in the first five years, whether after two weeks or after four years, is equally bad; at the same time, it ignores patient attitudes towards risk taking and the distinction between early death (for example perioperative mortality) and death from the disease itself."[22] In another study the same authors analyzed the value trade-offs in cancer of the larynx, finding that most people would sacrifice 15 to 30 percent of their normal life expectancy for better quality of life, choosing radiotherapy instead of laryngectomy. They conclude:

> This study has a straightforward message: Patients' attitudes toward morbidity are important, and survival is not their only consideration. Such attitudes vary enormously from patient to patient. These results seem to preclude paternalistic decisions based on "my clinical experience with patients who have your disease."[23]

Even if patients may not wish to make difficult decisions, their own best interests must be protected. In cases involving risk this requires asking patients about their values and factoring them into the decision. To strike a balance between risks and benefits in such decisions requires that both the physician's and the patient's values be made explicit.[24] Beck et al. now accept this view and approximate patient values about life expectancy and quality of life in a sophisticated analysis, saying, "We have found no substitute for a careful incorporation of patient attitudes into a clinical decision analysis."[25]

In this respect the doctor's first duty is to give patients sufficient information, not primarily for the sake of an "informed decision," which is very difficult in the face of various risks and uncertainities, but to help the patient discover and express his or her own values. When patients complain (one-half of 1,043 patients in one study)[26] that the information is unsatisfactory, it may be that information was complete and correct but not helpful because it did not assist patients in addressing their own values. This supposition requires more careful empirical verification than is now available.

An excellent example of the kind of decision making needed is provided by Schain's article about a woman's role in decisions regarding treatment of breast cancer. This is an example of decision making under risk since the probabilities are fairly well established for different treatment options. In a "fiduciary beneficence" model, for which we, too, have been arguing, the "physician *helps* the patient help herself." Schain states, "In the parlance of transactional analysis, this behavior is characterized by an 'adult-adult' communication with one member having specialized knowledge the other needs."[27] She rightly concludes that such a model promotes personalism rather than paternalism, unlike May, who is still concerned that a beneficence model detracts from patient autonomy by overemphasizing patient need.[28]

The third type of medical decision is decision under uncertainty, in which the outcomes are not or cannot be known, although some intermediate steps may be known. A classic description, also sensitive to patient values, is provided by Vaupel regarding a case published by Veatch. Ruth Mason, a client in genetic counseling, wants to know if she should have a child at risk for hemophilia. She must make five decisions: whether or not to have the carrier test, to become pregnant, to have amniocentesis, to abort, and later, to adopt. Vaupel argues that decision problems worth solving have no objective solution, and that "no real-life decisions can be made objectively." Subjective values enter such decisions at many points. They include which factors to consider, which past data may be used to refer to the future, which analyses may be left incomplete to simplify the decision tree, and, of course, which objective or subjective values will be used to measure the desirability of outcomes. Decision analysis in these cases does not indicate the right response; rather, the moral worth of an individual's judgment determines the moral worth of the decision.[29] Ruth Mason must grapple with possible, but unknown, outcomes. For instance, if she decides to become pregnant, what are the chances of having a hemophiliac son or a carrier daughter? Since the chance of the former is high, should she have amniocentesis? Does that mean she would abort if the child were male and had the disease or were just a carrier? Is abortion really moral in such a case, since hemophiliacs can lead fairly decent lives even though dependent on expensive medication?

Under these circumstances the responsibility of health care professionals to act beneficently is exceptionally high, especially since we live in a society of strangers. Patients must be able to expect from health professionals they do not know well, or at all, the greatest attention to their benefit. The opportunity to manipulate patients who must make decisions under uncertainty is immense. As Tversky and Kahneman show in their classic study of decisions made under uncertainty, an individual's preference is dependent upon the way a choice is framed. That is why people seem to violate the rules of logical consistency and coherent patterns of thought and action.[30] In general, people seem to analyze problems only in terms of short-range effects, without attention to the frame of reference. If one is asked to choose between saving one hundred out of four hundred people, or a 60 percent chance to save two hundred out of four hundred, a majority choose the first option. If the question is framed oppositely, diametrically opposite choices are made. One is asked to choose between letting three hundred out of four hundred people die, or having a 40 percent chance of letting two hundred people die. People choose the second option.

We can easily imagine the possibility of a genetic counselor putting options before persons such as Ruth Mason in such a way that the negative features of one possibility are subtly and unconsciously contrasted to the positive features of another. This possibility is especially important if the findings of Self about physician value systems are true. Self found that physicians and medical students claim to have an objective value system in which rules and norms guide conduct, but act contrary to this system when asked to solve clinical problems. Almost one-half of those surveyed judged that acts were right or wrong depending on the context.[31-33] This consistency underlines our new insistence that moral values be included in the decision matrix.

If decision analysis reflects the structure of doctor-patient judgments, then the three types of decisions we have described require a beneficence model. So far the discussion has assumed the patient has some capacity to engage in value discussions. Let us now consider two possible impairments of that capacity.

DECISION MAKING IN THE PRESENCE OF DEATH

The backdrop of every clinical decision is a kind of hope. That is why physicians dealing with terminal patients rarely, if ever, spell out the entire course of the disease in all its gruesome detail. Instead, each piece of that quite predictable course is taken discretely. This is done in order to support the quality of the patient's life. Hope is seen as an essential component of that quality, as well as of the decisions that must be made. This is true even though the chances of improvement are slim or nonexistent.

In risky or uncertain decisions that must be made by people who are dying or who face a lifelong debilitating illness ending in certain death, the usual backdrop of hope is lost. Reasonable assurance that one's life plans can be fulfilled is no longer available. In such cases there seems to be no reason to choose one or the other treatment because, no matter which decision is made, the outcome itself is certain. One will either die or face major personal disruptions of one's life plans. Though we still consider such persons free to make decisions and function as human beings, they are futureless. Since the future and hope are very much part of normal decision making, we must conclude that these persons are in a state of diminished humanity.

As a consequence they are even more vulnerable than other patients to the suggestions or recommendations of their physicians. This is especially true if they have been under the care of one physician for some time before having to make the decision in question. In such circumstances the principle of beneficence requires, if anything, the highest degree of compassion and sophistication about the patient's values, for these values must determine which decision will be made, even if the patient asks the doctor to decide and trusts the doctor's expertise.

It is tempting, in such cases, to grab hold of the only objective data we have—statistical date about effectiveness, five-year survival, and the like. Thus, Altman quotes Francis Galton's claim that statistics "are the only tools by which an opening can be cut through the formidable thicket of difficulties that bars the path of those who pursue the Science of man."[34]

Statistical analysis of data is essential to scientific research. It is less certain that these analyses can really provide the help patients need when they can make no long-term plans. These data concern longevity rather than quality of life, and it is here that statistics are not very helpful.

The first and most obvious reason for this difficulty is that much of what passes for "data" is not accurate. Because of bias in patient selection,[35] inadequate follow-up, and premature reporting, many studies may not be solidly grounded. Even in properly controlled studies, heterogeneous groups of patients may be entered—for example, patients having cancers in different stages or for different lengths of time, may be compared or patients who are ambulatory may be grouped with hospitalized ones who do only half as well. Further, the results of many studies are contradictory or unconvincing. Out of one hundred trials of radiotherapy for cancer in 1982, only twenty showed "results worthy of publication."[36] Furthermore, selection bias leads nonrandomized studies to be falsely optimistic or even wrong about new treatment.[37] Some studies have had too small a population to generate statistically significant data.

For these reasons, recommendations about treatments have to be made cautiously if we are not to violate the principle of doing no harm. There is also great dispute over methods of randomized or controlled clinical trials. In this dispute, not only scientific issues but also issues of beneficence are at stake. Let us look at a few examples.

Some radiotherapists argue that adjuvant radiotherapy for breast cancer does no good at all and, in fact, may cause later cancers. Others argue that the evidence for this claim does not exist or can be scientifically disputed. Still others point out that there is no improved survival rate for some breast cancers in any interventions compared with those left untreated. And, of course, everyone is familiar with the confusion about the evidence supporting a choice between lumpectomy, removal of a breast, or radical mastectomy. What statistics can actually be cited with certainty in order to help patients make decisions?[38,39]

In a study of bias in analytic research, 149 published research papers were examined and only 28 percent were judged acceptable by scientific standards. Fifty-six separate kinds of biases can enter clinical studies, rendering them invalid, It is hard to avoid making some mistakes in design, implementation, or interpretation.[40,41]

There is no way to assess the impact of unproven remedies in cancer therapy. Once patients perceive that doctors can do no more for them, they turn to a "cancer underground." A majority of patients never speak to their doctors about these remedies, but an impressive variety of fifty different ones are known to patients. About one-third of all cancer patients use them at one time or another during their regular therapy, and many of the patients in one study who did so were highly educated.[42,43] What impact does such lack of compliance have on the cancer data we possess?

There is currently a major dispute about the ethics of randomized clinical trials. Some objections have to do with design, some with interpretation, and some with the duty of physicians to act in the best interest of their patients.[44] For example, after a thirteen-year experience with aortacoronary bypass surgery, some investigators focused on whether or not the procedure saved or prolonged life. A much-publicized Veterans Administration cooperative study, a random-ized prospective trial, found no survival benefits from the operation. "Stuff and nonsense," De Bakey and Lawrie protested. They cited an astonishing near-nor-mal 90.4 percent 5-year crude survival rate in their series.[45] In other words, De Bakey and Lawrie claim that clinical experience, a time-tested method, was suf-ficient to determine the efficacy of a technique.

Given these sorts of problems with medical data regarding life-threatening diseases, the clinician's instinct to avoid using statistics in order to raise or dash a patient's hopes is sound. We do not mean to argue that disputes in science must vanish before we can use clinical data, but only that caution be exercised. These uncertainties reinforce our belief that patient values about chronic and debilitating disease should be the keystone treatment decisions about dying per-sons. For example, 33 percent of a surveyed group said they would accept a lifetime of hospital dialysis in order to stay alive; 68 percent of the same group would accept confinement at home to stay alive.[46]

If, in order to benefit their patients, physicians supply the hope that a serious disease destroys, then the use of statistical data and scientific results to decide on therapeutic intervention becomes a secondary concern. Statistical data can, within a jointly made decision, be used on a temporary basis until all parties involved concur that it is time to stop and permit the person to die; this time can generally be recognized by physicians, families, and patients. If the com-munication among them is good, there will be congruity because all will base the decision on benefit rather than on other standards. As can be seen, avail-ability of statistical data does not remove the requirement to make decisions on the basis of benefit to patients. Nor do data provide a mathematically sound index that can supplant the necessary value discussions between doctor and patient.

COMPROMISED COMPETENCE

Beneficence is also required in cases in which the decisions to be made are quite clear but the patient has either diminished or compromised competence. Such persons do not lack the freedom to act because they do not possess the means to do so (as do persons who lack knowledge, or, possessing knowledge, lack cer-titude about outcomes) but because they have an impaired power for reasoned choice. In such cases someone must act on the patient's behalf to respect his or her wishes, if they have been expressed.

Everyone can agree that in these circumstances a judgment is made about the quality of life. Patients who were once competent have a right to have their wishes about treatment respected, even if they have now lost one or another of the forms of competence (to make decisions, perform, or formulate life plans).[47] Although written in 1968, Symmers' description of a man not allowed to die is still pertinent today. In Symmers' account a sixty-eight-year-old doctor had metastatic cancer of the stomach. His pain was severe but only partially con-trolled by morphine. Ten days after hospitalization he suffered a pulmonary embolus, and a successful embolectomy was performed. He then made a written request not to be "saved" again. But fourteen days later he was rescued five times during cardiac arrest. He spent his last days decerebrate; on ventilation through a tracheostomy; and receiving intravenous fluids, blood products, antibiotics, and antifungal agents.[48] Presumably, someone in charge judged this dying doctor incompetent to make a judgment about his own treatment. Ignoring such a request to forego further treatment is a violation of both autonomy and beneficence.

The argument that illness destroys autonomy, and that beneficence or paternalism must therefore enter to fill the gap is now well developed. Disease may have one of the following three impacts on persons:

1. The disease disrupts the body in such a way that it leads to a reduced biological capacity.
2. The disease affects the patient's range of experience, leading to altered relations to the environment.
3. The disease is a severe threat to life and self-esteem.[49]

Simply being hospitalized causes stress and anxiety, not only about serious disease but also about not being told a diagnosis or the results of a test.[50] Illness, therefore, always distorts competence to make decisions that are in one's own best interests.[51-53] In this respect Cassell has expressed the now-classic position:

> When philosophers and lawyers (and many others) talk about rights they often speak as though the body does not exist. When they discuss the rights of patients they act as if a sick person is simply a well person with an illness appended. . . . that is simply a wrong view of the sick. . . . in the simplest terms, it is difficult to be clear-headed in pain or suffering. . . . Illness interferes with autonomy to a degree dependent on the nature and severity of the illness, the person involved, and the setting.[54]

Although these reflections do, indeed, lead directly to an argument that persons in a diminished state of competence need physicians and others to act on their behalf, it is important to recognize, as Baumgarten does, that sickness does not always impede a person's true wishes. Sickness may be what he calls "a transforming experience in a person's life," sometimes as profound as a religious conversion.[55]

To avoid the conclusion that everyone who is ill is incompetent and must therefore be treated until absolutely every avenue is exhausted, some criteria for stopping or withholding treatment are required. Some examples are brain death, a valid living will, and the opinions of a hospital ethics committee. On this matter Callahan proposes a definition of "natural death," namely, when one's life work is finished (just as a Beethoven sonata must come to an end), when one's moral obligations to others have been discharged, when one's death would not be seen as a moral outrage by others, and when one's dying is not marked by a process of unbearable and degrading pain. Callahan proposes these conditions to help us recognize the limits of efforts to conquer death or unduly prolong life.[56] But his proposal falls victim to an inherent contradiction between a "natural" end of life and a modern view of subjective self-fulfillment and individuality. In this view happiness resides not in attaining a goal or an end but in a restless pursuit of one goal after another.[47] In the latter view there is no "natural" end.

Because of the lack of unanimity on these approaches, a variety of criteria have been proposed. One is the substituted judgment standard, which may be interpreted in two ways: more commonly, as the decision the incompetent patient would make—using his or her own values—were she competent; less commonly, as the decision the surrogate would make were he or she in the incompetent patient's situation. The first construal is morally defensible; the second is less so because it assumes that someone else can judge the patient's best interests. When there is no knowledge at all of the patient's wishes, we may have to resort to the second meaning of substituted judgment.

Another criterion is McCormick's "reasonable person standard." Here one acts on behalf of others on the basis of what a community of persons of similar cultural, ethnic, and class backgrounds would find reasonable. This criterion avoids the dangers of capricious individual judgments by substituting the judgment of a community. One drawback is that introduces the danger of maleficence if it is applied to a patient from a community with values decidedly at variance with those of the community from which the "reasonable person" making the decision comes.

Finally, the durable power of attorney can be set. This is a legal instrument that empowers an individual to act on behalf of another without trying to anticipate all circumstances. The directions to the power of attorney may be detailed or general. They have both moral and legal force.

Instead, we prefer to honor the personhood of an incompetent patient by deciding what is in his or her best interest on the basis of what other patients like her, under similar conditions but competent, have tended to choose.[58] We agree with Cohen, who argues that some criterion is needed for the voiceless to ensure that they are not subject to a "life that denies all that is distinctively valuable about human beings."[59] Thus, the quality of life of others can be measured in terms of standards of individual well-being. It seems to us that Momeyer was groping toward a similar view, which he calls "situationally inferable judgment," as a form of best-interests criterion. This would mediate between respect for an autonomy that would be recklessly suicidal, on the one hand, and an undue burden on others, on the other.[60]

As we have pointed out, philosophers may mistake beneficence for paternalism. Thus, Gadow argues, "The benefit principle does not entail regard for autonomy, except perhaps when autonomy is subsumed under the category of benefit and is respected only when the professional deems it therapeutic; in theory the benefit principle assumes the waiving of autonomy."[61]

This statement is precisely what we deny. Acting for the best interests of others means acting on their behalf, in partnership with them, in order to help them. It requires sophisticated respect for independence of judgment and personal liberty. Autonomy, then, is not waived, as Gadow believes. In the case of incompetent persons, however, illness and incapacitation have already impeded it. Further, the choice of a criterion for making judgments about incompetent patients, even if that criterion is to be restoration of autonomy or respect for freedom of choice, itself depends on a judgment of what will best benefit the patient. Therefore, beneficence precedes autonomy in medical decision making.

We have shown that decisions made under uncertainty require particular attention to patient values and beneficence, what we call beneficence-in-trust. When utilities are calculated, they should include patient values. When these values are unknown due to incompetency, presumed wishes guide the practitioner. We will now turn to a more complete analysis of the clinical judgments made about the competency of patients.

12

Making Decisions for Incompetent Patients

Every clinical decision involves some assessment of the patient's competence—his or her capacity to make conscious and reasoned choices in matters relating to his own medical and health care. Competence is central to the moral validity of clinical decisions because competence is a necessary prerequisite to informed consent. Incompetence is a moral warrant for others to take actions they perceive to be in the patient's best interests, even against the patient's expressed wishes.

Informal assessments of competence are a daily responsibility of every physician. They are far more numerous than formal assessments made by psychiatrists, psychologists, judges, or courts. Indeed, they are the crucial and inescapable gateway to formal assessment, since only when competence is in doubt are the more formal procedures invoked.

Informal assessments do not differ in substance from formal assessments. They must address the same central question: Does *this* patient possess the capacity to make a conscious and reasoned choice at *this* time, in *this* context, and about *this* treatment? Informal assessments are therefore subject to the same ambiguity, complexity, possibility of error, and bias as formal assessments.

Informal assessments, in addition, have several characteristics that give them a special moral urgency. They are usually made privately by physicians and are not subjected to the usual formal scrutiny of formal determinations. Also, they are often made in situations of clinical urgency, in which neither physicians nor patients enjoy the advantages of deliberate and careful reflection. Finally, they are made by physicians not specifically trained to evaluate disor-

148

ders of mentation. It is these qualities—deliberateness, explicitness, and the expertise employed—that separate formal from informal assessments.

The importance of competency assessment and its relationships with autonomy, paternalism and beneficence, law, and psychiatry have generated a sizable literature, which this chapter will not attempt to analyze critically. Rather, our objective is to examine the conditions under which informal assessments are made, the way determinations of competence and incompetence relate to those conditions, and the moral guidelines, respecting beneficence-in-trust, that the general clinician should follow in making informal assessments. To attain these objectives we must examine some operating definitions of competence, the impediments to its operation, and the conditions under which informal assessments can be made correctly, objectively, and with as much moral sensitivity as possible.

THE COMPETENT PATIENT AND THE COMPETENT DECISION

The most widely accepted definition of competence is its identification as a capacity for performance of a specific task. In medical affairs the task in question is the limited one of making a reasoned choice among alternative courses of action presumed to benefit a sick person. A distinction can be made between a competent person and a competent decision. However, the exigencies of clinical decision making are best served by primary emphasis on the characteristics of a competent person, and only secondarily on the "competence" or "incompetence" of the decision itself.

A competent person possesses the capacity to make an explicit, reasoned, and intentional choice among alternative courses of action. At a minimum this capacity includes some substantial measure of the following capabilities: (1) The capacity to receive, comprehend, retain, and recall information provided by others or gathered by oneself. Information may be conveyed by word of mouth, writing, or some set of mutually understood set of signals. (2) The capacity to perceive the relationship of the information received to one's current clinical predicament as a sick person for whom something might or might not be done to cure, contain, or prevent illness or its symptoms. (3) The capacity to integrate and order the information received and to relate it to a realistic perception of the need for making a choice in such a way that the patient can weigh benefits and risks against some set of personal values. (4) The capacity to select an option, to give cogent reasons for the choice, and to persevere in that choice, at least until the decision is acted upon. (5) The capacity to communicate one's choice to others in an unequivocal manner. Among these capacities we include Culver and Gert's requirement that the patient understands the activity in question and knows when he or she is doing it.[1] This is implicit in the use of the term *conscious and reasoned choice* that is employed in this chapter.

A person possessing these capabilities should, other things being equal, be competent. A person lacking one or another of them is not necessarily incompetent. Whether competence should be a yes-or-no decision or whether it instead exists on a continuum is an arguable question. Wikler suggests two options: One is that competence is a matter of degree, that people possess more or less competence, and that the dividing line is a thin and arbitrary one. The other option is that there is a threshold for competence, and, once over that threshold, people will be equally competent to perform a given task, though their additional capacities beyond the threshold may differ substantially.[2]

Beauchamp and McCullough suggest that Wikler's dichotomy can be eliminated if "equally competent" is replaced by "sufficiently competent."[3] This seems a reasonable compromise since the empirical question is whether or not, in this instance, the patient is capable of a reasoned and conscious choice, not whether he or she can make the decision superlatively well.

One caveat, to which we shall refer later, is that it is important to avoid tying competence so closely to the nature of the decision that anyone not making the "right" decision in a given situation is considered insufficiently competent. A warning by the president's commission arises from clinical experience. Often patients are considered competent if they agree with the physician's recommendations, but are considered incompetent if they disagree or refuse to follow them.[4] Beauchamp and McCullough tend in this direction in their discussion of the concept of competence and criteria for intervention.[5] The distinction between competence and decisions is important because, in its absence, there is the danger of conflating the competence of the patient and the competence of his or her decision.

Whether one accepts the threshold or the relativistic conceptions of competence, the empirical assessment of competence depends upon criteria or tests that provide no absolute dividing line between competence and incompetence. The criteria used to measure competence and incompetence are external evidence of an interior capacity for conscious and reasoned decision and choice. The crucial empirical question is where to draw the threshold line or point on a continuous spectrum from unquestioned competence to unquestioned incompetence.

The criteria themselves, their validity, and their relationships to the criteria for autonomy are treated in more detail by other authors.[6] What is important here is that judgments of incompetence or competence are, in fact, made on the basis of the patient's possession of some threshold combination of capacities that are ascertainable by clinicians with varying degrees of certitude.

Possession of the threshold level of capabilities for competence does not mean these powers will, or necessarily can, be exercised. Various forms of coercion or duress, overt or covert, as well as insufficient or erroneous information, fear, anxiety, the pathophysiological accompaniments of illness—all can impede the operation of the capacities for competent judgments. But automatic declarations of incompetence based on the mere existence of one or more of these factors is unwarranted.

Possession of the capacities for competent judgment does not of itself assure informed consent. Informed consent implies both competence and autonomy, and adequate information and autonomy do not assure competence. There must also be the capacity to process information and to use freedom in a reasoned way.

Competence and autonomy are closely allied, and the criteria for determining each are closely interrelated. Suffice to say that they are not identical concepts. Incompetent patients may act autonomously—without external coercion, manipulation, or deception. Some competent patients, even under severe external duress, may retain their capacities for competent judgment and decision; others may not. Autonomy focuses on self-governance, the freedom to make one's own decisions; competence focuses on making one's own decisions in a reasoned and conscious way. Internal factors such as great fear, neurotic obsessions or compulsions, or drug addiction can impair both autonomy and competence.

Even in ordinary decisions, autonomy and competence are relative and their operation is difficult to evaluate. Most significant human decisions—to buy a house, to marry or divorce, or to take a new job—involve some degree of anxiety, fear, group or familial pressure, or threats to property, status, or finances. One sign of the capacity for competence is the ability to appreciate how these factors operate and how they should be weighed in making a decision.

We recognize that, even in the absence of illness, competence is not a global or permanent capacity. We recognize that we are competent for some tasks and not for others, and that at different stages of our lives we possess and lose our capacity for competence for some specific task. In the presence of serious illness, this propensity for selectively intermittent competence is exaggerated. The patient may be confused, disoriented, and senile, yet may be able to grasp the meaning and necessity of a limited immediate medical decision while lacking competence for larger decisions such as management of property or investments. Even the psychotic patient may be competent to make decisions about treatment.

Competence is a capacity; the decision is the product of that capacity. Yet one need not necessarily follow the other. Ordinarily, a patient capable of making conscious and reasoned choices can be expected to make a competent decision. The decision may be considered erroneous or harmful when it is not in conformity with the physicians's recommendations, with some external calculus of risks and benefits, or with the decision a "reasonable" person would make. But that does not, ipso facto, make the patient incompetent. On the other hand, a totally incompetent patient could make the "right" decision (that is, by agreeing with the medical recommendations) without the capacity for consciously reasoned choices.

When a competent patient makes a decision that may bring harm or death, that decision usually is the result of differences in the values or factual premises upon which it is based, or of an error in logic. For example, the patient may be given insufficient or erroneous information about a procedure or its risks and benefits. More often, the judgment that an otherwise competent patient has made an "incompetent" decision arises from differences in presuppositions about fundamental values of a religious or philosophical nature that, in the patient's life, take precedence over all other considerations. We might think that the patient's values are distorted, that we cannot in good conscience carry out his or her wishes, or that we ought, on paternalistic grounds, to intervene against the patient's choice. But disagreements at this level cannot justify labeling the patient as incompetent unless there is evidence of a defect in the capacity to make a reasoned decision.

The same applies to self-imposed constraints on freedom of choice. Roman Catholics are not free to participate in abortion or direct euthanasia; Orthodox Jews are not free to directly shorten a dying patient's life; a Jehovah's Witness is not free to accept a transfusion. Most humans have some set of self-imposed constraints that cannot legitimately be counted as evidence against either competence or autonomy. When the premises are empirically falsifiable, as with some psychotic patients, then they do constitute impediments to competent decision making.

Competence in the medical setting is the capacity for conscious and reasoned choices about one's own health and medical care. As a concept it is limited to the specific clinical instance. It is not global; it need not be permanent; it is judged by the capacity to make a consciously reasoned decision and not necessarily by the content of that decision. It is empirically tested by criteria based in an assessment of external signs of the operation of the internal capacity to make reasoned choices. These criteria measure the possession of some threshold level of capability beyond which a person is presumed to be sufficiently able to make his or her own decision, and to be permitted to do so.

COMPETENCY ASSESSMENTS IN ACUTELY ILL PATIENTS

All the uncertainties in the determination of competence and its empirical evaluation are compounded in acute illnesses and emergencies. In these circumstance physicians are confronted with urgent situations in which decisions must be made quickly, often without adequate information or preparation of the patient or the family. In addition, the illness or injury may be attended by pathophysiological disorders of mentation. Such disorders may result from pathological lesions in the brain itself, such as tumors, encephalitis, stroke, meningitis, brain contusion, or laceration. Or the primary source of disordered mentation may arise outside the brain, affecting its function temporarily—for example, anxiety, pain, shock, medications of all sorts, dehydration, azotemia, acidemia, electrolyte disturbances, hypoglycemia, anoxemia, or hypercapnia. The latter are often accompaniments of treatable disorders. They may impair brain function temporarily, but can often be reversed by appropriate therapeutic maneuvers.

Under these circumstances it is hardly imaginable that all of the detailed legal and philosophical criteria for assuring competent decisions can be fulfilled. The physician is caught between the duty of nonmaleficence, on the one hand, and respect for the patient's choice, on the other. How competent is a severely burned patient who asks not to be treated?[7] How competent is a patient with airway obstruction that causes severe anoexmia, hypercapnia, and acidemia? Or the patient with increased intracranial pressure who refuses, or for that matter, accepts, craniotomy?

Matters are further complicated when the acute episode is part of a chronic, recurrent, ultimately fatal disorder. In our view, beneficence-in-trust might presume in favor of overriding the patient's choice not to be treated in a first acute episode when the doctor knows little about the patient's values. The patient may recover from the first or subsequent episodes and then make a competent decision not to be treated. The patient may change his or her mind again when a new acute episode occurs. For example, a patient may ask, when not in acute distress, that vigorous resuscitative measures not to be used in her next episode. The decision may be made with doctor and family assenting, and it may be incorporated into a living will. The decision might fit the criteria for competency very well. Yet when the actual moment of decision arrives and the patient is bleeding acutely or unable to breathe, she may well ask that her decision be reversed. This has often happened to critical care physicians and is a source of great anxiety when it does occur.

There is usually little time in emergencies or acute illness for formal determinations of competence. Often the physician is forced to make the roughest kind of assessment. In addition to the inherent uncertainties, the decision may be influenced by the duress experienced by the physician. Decisions in acute emergencies are attended by urgency, confusion, and the distress of families and friends whose advice and information about the patient's wishes may be contradictory or inadequate. The physician may fear a malpractice suit or he or she may be an inexperienced resident.

Not all physicians are endowed with equanimity or objectivity that assures them of a capacity for conscious and reasoned judgments. The physician's duress may undermine two components of his or her own capacity for conscious reasoned judgment: assessing the patient's competency and making the technically correct decision. This is a factor that deserves some attention, since informal assessments of competence must sooner or later take into account the physician's psychological competence, as well as the patient's.

Several clinicians have examined the special difficulties of assessing both autonomy and competence in the actual clinical situation.[8,9] They underscore the factors that make these judgments difficult and uncertain, that influence the physician's decisions, and that diminish the patient's capacities for reasoned choice. Their central concern is for the conflict between the physician's traditional commitment to beneficence and nonmaleficence and the requirement to respect patient autonomy. Jackson and Youngner, and Siegler, like Childress, tie assessments of competence closely to what should be done in treating the incompetent patient.[10] While this is an important relationship, tying incompetence and intervention too closely slants the assessment of competence rather strongly in the direction of intervention.

Siegler, for example, proposes six factors that influence the physician's decision to respect the wishes of a critically ill patient: the patient's capacity to make a choice; the consistency of the choice with the patient's prior values; the patient's age; the treatability of the disease; the physician's value system; and whether the patient's decision is being made in the hospital, in the physician's office, or at home.[11] Of these six criteria only the first deals specifically with the patient's competence. The others concentrate on whether the decision the patient has made should be respected.

Thus, age is significant only if the patient is too young to be competent. But age is a relative matter since children mature at different rates, physically, intellectually, and psychologically. Many children under the legal age for independence can make competent decisions, while more than a few over that age cannot do so. This holds true for age in adulthood as well, though the presumption is always in favor of legal competence.

Consistency of the choice with the patient's prior or "true" value system is not relevant to competence assessment in the acute situation. Under such conditions the patient's values or prior assertions about what he or she would want done could change drastically. In the face of the immediate consequences of an earlier decision, the change may be in either direction, for or against treatment. Indeed, the patient may change his values several times, so that instability of values is not prima facie evidence of incompetence. The psychological stress and uncertainty of acute illnesses make vacillation and velleity the normal accompaniment of patient choices.

For similar reasons, Youngner and Jackson's identification of "true" autonomy with the choice the patient would have made were he or she in a calm and deliberate state is extremely dubious.[12] The patient is de facto *not* in a calm or deliberate state when he is making his choice. Few of us can predict what choices we, or others, might make when we actually experience the pain, discomfort, anxiety, and prospects of death an acute illness may present. These factors are part of the decision in acute illness. To take "true" autonomy out of the actual context of the decision is to abstract it from reality. Indeed, it may be a sign of true autonomy or competence to change one's mind about a theoretical choice in the face of the actual experience.

Some physicians take the state of illness itself to be an automatic impediment to competent decisions. They argue that the dependence of the sick person, the difficulties of understanding technical terms, and the need to trust the physician's judgment make competence and informed consent moot points. Some even assert, without compunction, that they can get any decision they want by the way they present the "facts." They assume that all patients are, in part, incompetent and that the physician therefore has a duty to manipulate the decision in the "right" direction.

The phenomenology of illness does, indeed, impose limitations on the patient's freedom in several domains. The sick person is forced to accommodate the demands of pain, disability, and anxiety. His or her body becomes a preoccupation and a central focus for conscious concern. The ill person is forced to depend on the knowledge, skill, and integrity of the physician, a person who can exert considerable power for good or evil. These facts make the relationship one of inequality, and the sick person is often forced by them into a vulnerable and exploitable state that is highly variable from one person to another.[13]

Though these features of illness do have an impact on autonomy, none of this justifies an automatic judgment of incompetence to make decisions. All decisions, clinical and otherwise, occur at bifurcation points in life and imply some degree of stress. The presence of obstacles to competence imposes a special obligation to remove them in order to enhance competence to the extent possible, and, thus, to restore the locus of decision making to the patient. To assume incompetence, or to place obstacles in the way of the patient's exercise of his or her capabilities for competent judgment (for example, deception or by provision of incomplete information) is a serious misconstrual of beneficence. It is, in fact, paternalism since it impedes rather than enhances patient choices.

The treatability of illness, even its gravity, should not predetermine the assessment of competence since the question is whether the patient wants treatment, not whether he or she needs it. Similarly, the place in which the decision is made—home, office, or hopsital—may condition how the decision about competence is made but does not affect the patient's competence.

The physician's own values, finally, are relevant only if the decision of a competent patient conflicts with the physician's conscience so that he or she feels unable to or cannot cooperate with it. As already pointed out, disagreement with the physician's recommendations is not a final criterion of competence.

Siegler's criteria are a more accurate reflection of the criteria physicians actually use in decisions to intervene than of criteria employed in decisions about competence. There is some justification to further use on the grounds of clinical discretion.[14] But clinical discretion does not vitiate the importance of keeping decisions about the patient's competence separate from those about interventions against his will. The patient's best interests, as a rational and sentient being, are better served by making these judgments in separate steps, related to, but not telescoped into, one another.

AUTONOMY AND BENEFICENCE IN COMPETENCE ASSESSMENT

Despite the physician's best efforts to make competency assessment as objective as possible, value desiderata will intrude themselves. They cannot be eliminated as long as medicine remains an interaction of persons. Beauchamp and McCullough underscore how strongly value presuppositions may condition the stringency with which physicians apply the criteria or competence.[15] They call for clearer reasoning to deal with the potential conflicts that may arise between the principles of beneficence and autonomy at the moment of clinical decision.

This is certainly a necessary step. But reasoning alone will not resolve deeper conflicts of values since they arise in a conflict of axioms rather than a conflict of logic. The key question is which should be the dominant principle— the patient's freedom to choose what he or she thinks is good, or the doctor's freedom to intervene when, in his or her opinion, the patient has made a harmful or dangerous choice? Roth and his coworkers try to resolve this matter by relating their criteria of competence to the gravity and consequences of the decision to be made. When the decision involves a treatment that could save the patient's life—for example, transfusion in severe blood loss—they would recommend that the more stringent criteria for competence be applied. When the decision is of a less definite nature—for example, treating arthritis—they allow for a much looser interpretation.[16] This is not unlike our earlier assertion that healing is the goal of the doctor-patient relation, and that this value is non-negotiable if healing is to take place. Roth et al. assume this is the purpose of interventions on the patient's behalf.

But this solution as applied to competency has several shortcomings. First of all, it reinforces the relativistic character of competence assessment. It increases the likelihood of fitting competency assessment to the physician's values and puts the patient's autonomy at considerable risk by giving too easily an automatic warrant for medical intervention over the patient's wishes.

Another shortcoming is the presumption that beneficence is synonymous with strong or weak paternalism. As we have argued, beneficence can also be interpreted as acting in such a way as to enhance the patient's autonomy since autonomy is, itself, one level of good (see chapter 8). In this view we do harm to the patient if we override patient autonomy by declaring him or her incompetent in the truly important decisions outlined by Roth et al. These considerations take us back inevitably to the need for clarification of our conceptions of beneficence, autonomy, and the patient's good. These crucial questions are obfuscated by assessments of competence that are situation-dependent. Such assessments beg the question by presuming that when the patient disagrees with the doctor, "beneficence" (actually, paternalism) requires that autonomy be violated.

It seems preferable to consider competence as a capacity of the patient to be judged independently of the gravity of the decision, the doctor's recommendations, or of what a reasonable person would choose. The first step is to determine, as objectively as possible, whether the patient is competent. If the patient is judged incompetent, then we must face the next question: What moral warrant do we have for intervention against his choice?

This approach forces us to think more rigorously about imposing a choice on a competent patient. We cannot hide the decision behind a situation-dependent scale of competence. The light of argument, therefore, must be focused where it belongs—on the conflict between the fundamental values of beneficence and autonomy and on the need for a more holistic view of the good of the patient.

There is one aspect of intervention that is so closely tied to competence determination that it cannot be neatly separated from it. We refer to interventions designed to remove remediable causes of incompetence, such as ventilatory therapy to treat anorexia or hypercapnia, restoration of fluid and electrolyte balance, dialysis of azotemic patients, discontinuance of toxic drugs, or treatment of infection. Under these circumstances the physician is acting to restore competence so that the patient may participate in decisions that effect his well-being. In so doing he is acting paternalistically but in a morally defensible way.

Beauchamp and McCullough propose a graded system of justifications for intervention based upon the degree of reversibility of competence (and autonomy).[17] They give precedence to autonomy when competence is restorable and when a "value history" is available. They give precedence to beneficence when autonomy is irreversibly lost. Their system would accord roughly with the hierarchical ordering of patient good that we proposed in chapter 8.

We disagree, however, with Beauchamp and McCullough's contention that treatments aimed at restoring autonomy or competence should not be undertaken in the incompetent patient if he gave prior instructions against such treatments.[18] Our disagreement is limited to the case of the severely and acutely ill patient. Empirically, we all too often find with such patients that a prior request against specific treatments is reversed when the complete exigencies of rejection are fully comprehended. Beauchamp and McCullough seem to allow for some relaxation of their rule of freedom over beneficence in acutely ill patients. These are just the situations we have concentrated on in this chapter—those in which the opportunity for a "relaxed philosophical inquiry," as they put it, is impossible.[19]

It seems better from the standpoint of beneficence-in-trust to develop what we would call rules of clinical intervention. According to these rules, the larger goals of beneficence would permit the physician's intervention to restore competence and, in some cases, quality of life, even in the absence of consent or competence. In effect, these rules justify necessary medical paternalism. There are at least three rules, or three versions of the same rule:

1. *Weak form.* The least obtrusive form of the rule of clinical intervention is one in which reversing incompetence is possible. The rule might go as follows: The physician should always intervene to reverse potentially reversible conditions impeding competence. This should be done in spite of currently expressed wishes to the contrary since these wishes are now subject to the informal (and later, formal) judgments of incompetence. As noted earlier, such as intervention would not, strictly speaking, be a form of paternalism since it violates no moral rule. One acts in the best interests of the patient by overcoming an impediment. Of course, once competence has been reestablished, beneficence-in-trust requires honoring the competent wishes of the patient.

2. *Intermediate form.* More obtrusive, clearly paternalistic action might be justified in emergencies in which the extent of the injury and its implications for survival and quality of life are not yet known. This rule runs as follows: Physicians should always act to reverse trauma or illness in spite of contrary expressions until the condition is judged irreversible and hopeless, or until the patient's current wishes are demonstrated as antedating this new event and perduring to the present.

Once the condition or accident becomes a hopeless injury to the body, physicians should act in the best interests of their patients by withdrawing the life-supporting measures that are unduly prolonging dying. Since no reversibility is possible, emergency interventions (cardiopulmonary resuscitation, respirators, antibiotics, and so on) now become, in effect, instruments of suffering and pain since they merely prolong a dying process begun outside the walls of the hospital. The basis for stopping treatment is the previously expressed wish of the patient, which might have been temporarily ignored during the first stages of the emergency intervention. The only justification for continuance would be the preservation of organs for transplant. In any event, this justification always occurs after the patient has suffered brain death.

3. *Hard form.* The third rule of clinical intervention applies particularly to psychiatry and is most clearly a form of necessary medical paternalism. It has an analogue in pediatrics as well, as Ackerman has argued.[20] It reads as follows: The physician should always intervene to attempt reversal of psychiatric disorders which impede the patient's capacity to function as a person or social being (for example, severe depression limiting mobility) even if the patient has not been judged legally incompetent.

The hard form differs from the previous two forms of clinical intervention. First, the grounds for ignoring or overriding the wishes of a patient are a good, improved social functioning, rather than necessarily a restoration of competence. In this way a person with impaired competence, even if not severe enough to have him or her declared legally incompetent, would receive treatment the physician judged might improve her ability to deal with her impairment. To use our example, if a patient were so depressed that she could not leave her own living room, the physician could act to adjust drug dosages or apply electroconvulsive therapy without consent if there were reason to assume that the adjustment or treatment would improve the patient's capacity to function.

A second way in which this rule differs from the others is that it acts on psychological conditions that impede the capacity for social life rather than merely on physical conditions that obstruct competence. Like the other two rules, however, this one violates informed consent in favor of more important goods.

On the surface, the rules of clinical intervention seem to violate a fundamental principle of self-determination in their attempt to maintain the fiduciary model we have advanced. Thus, Mill noted in 1859 that "over himself, his own body and mind, the individual is sovereign."[21] In *Schloendorff v. The Society of New York Hospitals* (1914), Justice Cardozo's opinion stated, "Every human being of adult years and of sound mind has a right to determine what shall be done with his own body."[22] In *Natanson v. Kline* (1960), the court reaffirmed this principle, stating: "Each man is considered to be master of his own body and may, if he be of sound mind, prohibit the performance of life-saving surgery or other medical treatment."[23] Recent court cases such as *In re Bartling*[24] also confirm this legal doctrine, as did the president's commission, which upheld the right of competent patients to decide for themselves, even if refusal would lead to a premature death.[25]

Our proposed rules would not negate this tradition, even if that were possible. Instead, they deal with that "gray area" between competence and legally declared incompetence, the informal judgments of incompetence we have discussed in this chapter. In the weak form the patient has not been declared incompetent, but a temporary condition contributes to the informal assessment of incompetence. In the intermediate form a serious new event has affected the patient. While its reversibility is not as certain as is that of the weak form, it also contributes to an informal judgment of incompetence. Since it is not certain that the patient's previous refusal of therapy foresaw this new event (for example, refusal of the respirator in anticipation of a slow death from cancer), the refusal can be overridden until the crisis resolves or its seriousness is assessed. In the hard form we recognize the special case posed by psychiatric disorders that impede patient judgment even when the patient has not been declared incompetent. Many cases involve depressed patients whose medications require adjustment, often to a lower dose. For the purpose of medical treatment, they should be treated as one would treat an adolescent.

By proposing a rather strict set of rules governing the informal judgments of incompetence, and by basing these rules on the seriousness of the physical or mental disease that affects the patient, we avoid a sliding scale of criteria for incompetence based on the seriousness of the decision.[26]

SOME MORAL GUIDELINES FOR INFORMAL ASSESSMENT OF COMPETENCE

Granting the difficulties of informal assessments of competence, there seem to be some guidelines for making morally defensible competence assessments. To propose a set of guidelines requires some statement of the antecedent ordering principles on which they are based. The ordering principle should be the principle of beneficence, so interpreted that preservation of autonomy becomes a component of the patient's good and therefore consistent with, and not in opposition to, benevolence and beneficence.

Even in complex and urgent clinical situations, therefore, the nonpsychiatric physician should adhere to some explicit set of criteria of competence to the degree the clinical exigencies permit. He has a duty, therefore, to become particularly skillful in informal assessments of the disorders of mentation that may signal incompetence.

This is, incidentally, a neglected aspect of physicians' training, in which the usual assumption is that medical good overrides all other good in the care of seriously ill patients. As guardians of the gateway to more formal assessment, general clinicians must be able to evaluate the possibility that a patient may not be competent to make reasoned choices. The physician should then seek formal assessment through consultations.[27] If there is not enough time for a more formal assessment of psychological competence, the clinician must act so that whatever competence the patient possesses is utilized or enhanced in making decisions.

A particular responsibility of nonpsychiatrists is to evaluate as objectively as possible all those pathophysiologic or pathological conditions that can affect brain function and mentation, and therefore the capabilities needed for competent decisions. The physician and his or her colleagues need this information when making informal assessments, as does the psychiatric consultant in making a formal assessment. The clinician must also ascertain which of the impediments to competent decision making are reversible, and to what degree, and which are not.

The clinician has an obligation to enhance whatever degree of competence is present by treating reversible disorders of cerebral function. When this is accomplished, competence must be reassessed and the patient's choices restored to preeminence in decision making. In treating a reversible pathophysiological distrubance, the physician may override the objections of the patient unless the patient, before becoming incompetent, clearly, explicitly, and recently asked that such measures not be used. But even in these instances, if there is any doubt at all, competence should be restored to allow for as autonomous and as competent a set of subsequent decisions as possible. Note, however, that the physician must be prepared to stop treatments inaugurated earlier, if the patient so desires.

When patients wax and wane in their competence, and vacillate in their decisions for or against treatment, the last substantially competent decision should prevail. This will often be the case in chronic illness marked by acute exacerbations. Velleity and vacillation are not warrants for an automatic diagnosis of incompetence. The most recent competent wish of the patient should always be respected.

The physician must provide the patient or his or her proxy with the information necessary to make an informed and competent choice. Suffice it to say that the information should be provided without deception, coercion, or manipulation. The information also must be presented sensitively, in a way geared to the patient's capacity for understanding, to his education, and to his linguistic, cultural, and social milieu. This element of competent decision making is very much under the physician's control. For that reason, the physician has a moral obligation to take special pains in informing both the patient and the family. He must avoid the all-too-frequent judgment that a patient cannot comprehend the issue because it must be couched in technical language.[28].

When dealing with the proxy consent of family, friend, or legal guardian, the physician has an obligation to satisfy himself that the proxy is competent to make a choice for this patient, and that no conflict of interest with the good of the patient exists. If the proxy choice conflicts with the good of the patient, the physician's first obligation is to his patient. He is not bound automatically to accept a proxy decision.

When the physician finds the choice of a competent patient, or of the proxy, offensive to his or her own moral principles, the physician should withdraw from the case without endangering the patient's clinical outcome. He need not seek out another physician who will agree with the patient if he believes that the patient's choices involve a serious breach of morality (for some physicians, suicide or abortion). It is the responsibility of the physician to ascertain the competent patient's values and preferences before entering the new therapeutic relationship. The value history, the values patients have used in making important decisions in thier lives—medical or otherwise—should be part of the patient's initial history. This becomes increasingly important to preserve both the principles of autonomy and beneficence.

In all of this the assessment of competence should be made as objectively as possible, and should be distinct from the gravity of the decisions to be made or how to deal with the patient who is judged to be competent. Obviously, these domains must be related to each other, but in stepwise and modular fashion, not by blurring the distinctions between them. Furthermore, what we have noted about incompetent patients also applies to assessments of patients' parents, other family members, proxies, and guardians, a matter discussed in the next chapter.

If the patient's capacity for conscious reasoned choice is truly impaired, it should be so judged and the appropriate steps should be taken to protect his or her interests—whether or not the choice is serious. All the difficulties of making competency assessments stressed here are compounded by the fact that the defintion of "competence" is not clear.

Informal assessments of competence are the everyday business of every physician. They require a more explicit formulation than is now customary because competence is so central to informed consent, decisions to intervene in the patient's behalf, and protection of the patient's best interests.

We have mentioned the role of the family in decisions about incompetent patients and must explore this problem in the next chapter, defending some of the assertions made herein in greater detail.

13

The Role of Physicians, Families, and Other Surrogates in Decisions Concerning Incompetent Patients

In this book we have argued that the good of the competent patient is best served if, within certain limits, the patient is allowed to make decisions about what care he or she shall or shall not receive. We have described the hierarchy of goods that should guide both the patient and the physician in their choices. We have called for beneficence-in-trust to balance the tendency to absolutize patient autonomy as well as physician paternalism.

In this chapter our intent is to show how beneficence-in-trust functions in the more difficult situation of caring for the incompetent patient. When the capacity for reasoned choice is compromised or lost entirely, the patient is extremely vulnerable and even exploitable. Physicians, families, and other surrogates are tempted to move into the vacuum and give their personal interpretations of what the patient "really" would have wanted.

Under these circumstances the physician has a special obligation to act as steward of the patient's moral right to have his or her wishes fulfilled. This is not a moral warrant for the physician to impose his or her own values or make medical good the sole ordering principle. Nor does it mean slavishly and uncritically submitting to the surrogate's decisons. Rather, the obligation of that stewardship is to clarify, validate, and enhance the patient's will to the extent possible.

In the fulfillment of her stewardship function, the physician must enter into dialogue with a variety of proxies and surrogates, whether family members or not, and must try as best she can to interpret the patient's intent. Often she will encounter conflicts among surrogates' decisions, anticipatory declarations, family members, and other medical attendants.

How are these conflicts to be resolved in some morally defensible way? We propose a series of hierarchically arranged steps (based on those found in chapter 6) and an order of moral priority that, we believe, coincides with the guiding principle of beneficence-in-trust as we have tried to elucidate it:

1. the anticipatory declarations of the patient
2. the validated decisions of morally valid surrogates (e.g., family, friends, guardians, a durable power of attorney)
3. the physician
4. ethics committees
5. the courts

In each case the moral priority of the source of decisional authority depends on the ethical validity of the preferred decision; this, in turn, centers on its degree of fidelity to the patient's own values and belief systems.

ANTICIPATORY DECLARATIONS

An anticipatory declaration is an advance directive about health care.[1] It is an effective way for patients to anticipate certain events in the course of their illness or even long before they become ill, while still competent, in order to guide their families and medical attendants on such matters as when to withhold or withdraw certain forms of treatment or how vigorously to pursue other marginal treatments. The legal requirements of such wills vary from one state jurisdiction to another. This is not the place to discuss what constitutes a legally valid anticipatory statement. Rather, we are concerned here with the moral criteria for such statements, which are described below.

The statement must be free of coercion and must be made when the patient is competent. The patient must also realize that he or she may have, or actually has, an incurable condition. Just how long before this realization occurs such an anticipatory statement must be made is an open question, but it is a matter that must be examined to avoid carrying out instructions that might have been made capriciously or without sufficient thought. The most effective check would be to encourage anticipatory statements at any time in life and to ask the patient to reaffirm them when the terminal nature of his illness becomes manifest, but before coma or disordered states of mentation supervene.

Obviously, anticipatory statements must not have been made under coercion, on the basis of erroneous prognostications, or as a result of manipulation by the physician, the family, or others.[2]

Anticipatory declarations must be consistent with the patient's lifelong value system. Of course, patients can change those values when facing terminal illnesses, but when this occurs, the obligation to clarify and validate such a change is particularly strong.

Anticipatory statements also must be validated and given relative weights. Written declarations have more weight than oral ones, specific orders more weight than general admonitions, recent statements more than distant, repeated exhortations more than single instances, and those given in the absence of emotional stress more than those given in moments of depression.

Even if anticipatory declarations meet the criteria of moral validity, the physician has an obligation to enter into dialogue with the family or others who know the patient well. Few living wills or other prior statements can be so specific that they cover all clinical eventualities. The patient may have asked not to become a "burden" to his family. But what counts as a burden for one family may not be one for another. The patient may have asked that he not be intubated, force-fed, or placed on mechanical respirators, or that "extraordinary" measures not be used. It is important to be sure of what the patient understood these measures to mean. Some sense of the patient's comprehension and his lifelong values—that is, his "value history"—is essential to properly interpret his wishes.

This emphasis on clarification and validation of anticipatory declarations is not intended to make the physician the final judge. Rather, it is to require that he assure himself that he is indeed carrying out the patient's wishes as closely as possible. The physician must guard against the "Pontius Pilate syndrome"—washing his hands of responsibility because someone else claims to know the patient's wishes or because he has the legal sanction of a living will. As always, the physician is bonded to the patient, whose expectation is that the physician will be his agent and not someone else's.

SURROGATE DECISION MAKERS

In the absence of a morally valid anticipatory declaration, the physician turns to those who might be best able to substitute for the patient's judgment—that is, to make the decision the patient would have made were he or she able to do so. The surrogate may be the family, a friend, an acquaintance, someone with permanent power of attorney, or a legal guardian.

Some have argued that the family is almost always the best surrogate because of the family member's "bonding" to the patient.[3] This may not always be the case. The physician's first responsibility, as in the case of anticipatory declarations, is to ascertain the moral validity—that is to say, the moral acceptability—of the surrogate decision maker. This is the only way the physician can fulfill his or her own responsibility as steward of the patient's interests.

The criteria for a morally valid surrogate decision are as follows:

1. First, the surrogate must provide some evidence that he or she really knows the patient and his or her values. This is not necessarily the case even with families. In our mobile society parents and children are often separated geographically; they may be estranged from each other, or may not have seen each other for a long time. Friends may have a closer, or more recent, knowledge of what the patient would want. Nurses may know more about a patient in a long-term care setting than does the patient's family.

2. Further, the surrogate or proxy must not have a conflict of interest with

the patient's best interests. The desire for gain—settlement of an estate, inheritance of property, changing a will, and so on—can impel surrogates, consciously or not, to hasten a patient's death by undertreatment.[4]

3. Also to be guarded against is the deleterious effect of psychological antipathies—the unconscious desire to overtreat a patient whom one has neglected or maltreated for many years, or, conversely, the motivation to undertreat and thus act vindictively to settle old scores.

These impediments to surrogate decisions that genuinely reflect the patient's interests must be taken into consideration by the physician. Under the principles of beneficence-in-trust that we have been urging in this book, the physician has an obligation to be the patient's advocate. It is the physician, then, who must be reasonably sure that the surrogate is indeed making a morally valid substituted judgment.

Needless to say, if, by the criteria above, the patient has executed a morally valid anticipatory declaration or intention, such a statement takes moral precedence over the immediate wishes of the family. This may result in a serious conflict that can be settled only by a hospital ethics committee or, barring that, in a court action.

In the case of a durable power of attorney, the situation is in one sense simplified since another person has been empowered by the patient to make all decisions once the patient becomes incompetent. Such a person has a wide latitude to adapt to the specifics of a particular decision. But a person so empowered might nonetheless not always act in the patient's behalf. Everything considered, a durable power of attorney is as full an expression of confidence as one person can give another, and, except for the most serious reasons—such as obvious incompetence of the surrogate—the decision of the person granted this power ought to be followed.

The decision of legal guardians has less moral weight. Those who hold this authority for minors, the mentally retarded, or the aged may have only tenuous bonding with those they represent. In particular, conflicts of interest must be guarded against. The physician may well have to resist, and ask for court relief, when he or she thinks that the value system of the legal guardian is being imposed on the patient or that the decision of the guardian is not in the best interest of the patient. Pediatricians, especially, are enjoined by law, and are given appropriate powers to ensure that guardians make decisions in the best interests of a minor child.

The same conditions of moral validity apply in the case of the guardian ad litem, appointed by the court to protect and act for the incompetent patient in a particular circumstance. As difficult as the consequences may be, legal procedure cannot excuse the obligation of beneficence with which the physician is entrusted if serious harm threatens the patient. The guardian ad litem and the judge who appoints him or her have their own value systems, which may conflict with those of the incompetent patient. For this reason, the physician must be critical even of the legally appointed guardian of her patient since she, too, has a guardianship—one that is moral rather than legal.

What we are asserting, for both anticipatory declarations and surrogate decisions, is that priority must be given to the patient's wishes and that the physician has a responsibility to take reasonable measures to assure that anticipatory declarations and surrogate decisions are authentic. Since the physician is inescapably the agent who must carry out the surrogate decision, she must be certain that she is not cooperating with an immoral act.[5]

In this view the obligation to guard the patient's moral right to make her own decision is better grounded in the idea of informed consent than in the notions of autonomy or privacy. The latter have been the bases generally used by the courts. They can be traced back to Mill and to Justice Cardozo.[6] This, too, is the spirit of the recommendations of the President's Commission for the Study of Ethical Problems in Medicine and Biomedical and Behavioral Research.[7]

In our view the patient's wishes can be adequately respected only if the surrogate and the physician can make a genuine assessment of the patient's values in light of the context of choices this decision entails. When the patient is fully competent, this assessment requires a dialogue between physician and patient in which the physician makes an effort to examine the consistency of the present decision with the patient's fundamental values (which we distinguish from current preferences). Preferences are more apt to be ephemeral and hence should not be followed blindly when they seem inauthentic—that is, inconsistent with the patient's characteristic and expressed value system (if this is known).

This is not to suggest that what the physician judges to be a preference can by that mere fact be overridden. Rather, it argues for a sufficient dialogue between physician and patient to assure that a particular clinical decision or moral choice has the authenticity which the moral obligation to respect persons requires. Given this point of view, we prefer models of the physician-patient transaction that call for dialogue, dialectic, and consent; these include Siegler's accommodation model,[8] the therapeutic alliance of Jonsen, Siegler, and Winslade,[9] and the revised paternalism of Weiss.[10]

When the patient is incompetent, this dialogue is manifestly impossible. In a sense, however, the patient's anticipatory statement opens up a dialogue before the fact, but one in which the conscientious physician can ascertain the patient's wishes and distinguish her fundamental values from her preferences.[11] This dialogue serves to clarify for both patient and physician, at a time when the crisis of making a decision is not so overwhelming, what guidelines the patient wishes the physician to follow when crises do, in fact, arrive.

This view rests more explicitly on the physician's duty of beneficence than on autonomy as an absolute principle. Indeed, as the patient's illness progresses, her autonomy may be progressively compromised. In an overwhelming emergency there is neither time nor circumstance for the clarifying dialogue. The physician's presumption should be in favor of treatment until the patient or family have had sufficient time to place the required decisions within the context of the patient's wishes and values.

It would be dangerous for a rescue squad, for instance, to acquiesce in refusals of treatment, general or specific, at the roadside or in the home. Families and patients may be in conflict over whether or not a patient with a terminal disease should be treated or go to the hospital. But this is too complex a disagreement to be resolved simply on the basis of the patient's autonomous statement.

Of course, if the physician is present and knows the patient and her prior wishes, she could and should comply. But absolute respect for autonomy is too much of a moral burden to impose upon emergency medical personnel whose knowledge of the patient is necessarily sketchy and who must act in the midst of emotionally charged circumstances. In such situations the presumption must be for treatment for the emergency, leaving the finer decision about continuing treatment for a later time. In order for this approach to carry continued validity, however, health care professionals must be better able to withdraw treatment later than is presently the case.

THE PHYSICIAN AS SURROGATE AND ADVOCATE

When no morally valid surrogate or anticipatory declaration is available, or when the emergency is so acute that there is no time to consult them, the physician is forced into a triple role—as possessor of medical knowledge, as advocate, and as surrogate for the patient. Each role has moral obligations, and each may conflict with the others. The physician must recognize the obligations of each role, distinguish them clearly from each other, and put them in some order of priority. The criteria the physician uses should be consistent with beneficence-in-trust.

Under circumstances of incompetence and lack of evidence about values, the only level of the patient's good that is ascertainable with any degree of certitude is the medical good—what can be achieved by curing, containing, or ameliorating the disease. Some would interpret this to mean that, in the absence of instruction to the contrary, the physician is impelled to treat vigorously until the patient expires. In our view this is not consistent with beneficence since many treatments are futile, burdensome, expensive, and only prolong the act of dying. To rely solely on medical indications is to abnegate the advocate and surrogate roles that the circumstances thrust upon physicians.

If the physician feels, for reasons of conscience, unable to withhold or withdraw treatment, we believe that beneficence forces him or her to transfer care to another physician. If, on the other hand, the physician feels that under certain circumstances life support can be discontinued, then he must be clear about the moral validity of those circumstances.

This means that medical indications must be tempered by some construction of probable values the patient might be presumed to hold. This construction is not as arbitrary as it may first appear. Following the principle of beneficence-in-trust, the treatment should somehow benefit the patient. To do so it must be effective in either curing or containing the pathophysiologic processes, easing pain, or otherwise providing comfort. Also, the treatment should be beneficial as well as effective—that is, it must serve some interest of the patient. To treat pneumococcal pneumonia in a patient in a terminal state with malignant disease is an effective treatment, but not a beneficial one. The medical good—eliminating the infection—does not result in any good to the patient, but merely prolongs the act of dying.[12]

Even if a treatment is beneficial and effective, it must not be so burdensome that the benefits are outweighed.[13] Repeatedly reinserting a nasogastric or gastrostomy tube in a terminal, confused, and dying patient does not, on the face of it, offer any benefit. Although he or she may have asked that "everything be done," it is doubtful that even a competent patient would want to be assaulted daily to maintain hydration for the last days of life with no purpose other than prolonging life for a short time.

Care must be exercised to stay close to the notion of beneficence and to distinguish it from the usual quality-of-life criteria. We are concerned that the criteria of benefit, effectiveness, and burdens be related to the patient's physical and existential condition, and not to the place or utility of the patient in society (see chapter 7). Our concern is that we do no harm to the patient; thus, it is necessary to avoid therapeutic belligerence and meddlesome medicine—sustaining life at all costs even when, in the best clinical judgment, treatment is futile, burdensome, or of marginal benefit.

Two examples of therapeutic obstinacy will illustrate the point. In one instance we know of a dying cancer patient who was resuscitated twenty-one times in twenty-four hours. In another case a seventy-year-old woman with amotrophic lateral sclerosis was connected to a respirator when she suffered cardiac arrest, despite prior statements to family and friends that she did not want to be so treated. An out-of-town doctor had to be engaged and given hospital staff privileges so that, six months later, the respirator could be discontinued.[14]

In each of these instances, the physician's values were inimical to the patient's best interests. In each case the beneficence-in-trust model that we have been elaborating was violated. In this sense the physicians violated their guardianship of the patient's welfare even though they no doubt acted out of their own beliefs that to discontinue treatment would be morally wrong.[15]

Recall, that, in this circumstance, the morally conscientious physician has two valid choices. He may withdraw respectfully from the case or, if he believes a direct, serious harm is being done to the patient, he may have recourse to the court.

One of the difficulties with placing the physician third in the hierarchy of decision makers is that, given the impersonality of the modern health care system and, in some, the tendency to therapeutic belligerence, the physician may not be the best judge of what is best for the patient. Does our view require the physician's decision to dominate over that of family members? Our thesis is that the physician must husband the patient's known, presumed, or constructed (with the family) values and current preferences, not his own set of values. Then the judgment about the patient's best interests becomes a sophisticated balancing of the patient's values and a proportionate sense of the impact of medical interventions on that patient's condition. In this balancing the physician's special expertise is an essential, necessary, but not sufficient ingredient.

HOSPITAL ETHICS COMMITTEES

Conflicts that arise among the participants in clinical decisions may be of various origins—different interpretations of a patient's prior statements about treatment, the meaning of the terms of an anticipatory declaration, the weight that should be given to evidence of the patient's desires, questions of legality, conflicts between family members, or fundamental differences about the meaning and value of human life. Some of these differences might be resolved by recourse to an ethics committee. Among the several functions of these committees, which are gaining wide acceptance in hospitals in the United States, is the consultative and counseling role.[16] Here the party in conflict can obtain the benefit of opinions of others who are not immediately involved, professionally or emotionally, in the decision. By a careful examination of the issues, some of the differences no doubt can be resolved, or some negotiated agreement can be reached on what should be done.

Ethics committees do not decide moral issues. Their opinions do not bind the parties in a dispute. They especially do not resolve fundamental substantive ethical differences. However, properly used, they can defuse some of the emotional stress of difficult decisions. They are particularly valuable as buffers between the disputants and the courts, but they must be used sparingly and discriminantly. As Siegler points out, they should not substitute for bedside decisions.[17] Even if they could, the time required by committees to meet and discuss a case properly militates against their routine use.

The literature on ethics committees is expanding rapidly. Most hospitals are just becoming familiar with their use and are assessing their utility. We mention them here in order to locate them in the series of steps that can be taken to resolve serious conflicts about what is in a patient's best interest.

USE OF THE COURTS

When the patient's anticipatory declarations, the decision of morally valid surrogates or physicians acting in a surrogate capacity, or the use of ethics committees fails to result in decisions about the best interests of the incompetent patient, recourse must be had to the courts. In democratic societies the courts are the last resort for the resolution of otherwise irreconcilable disputes. The courts provide a "coarse" adjustment but a necessary one, without which decisions and actions might not occur, or the rights of the participants to a dispute might not be protected.

Like ethics committees, courts do not settle the moral issue. Their emphasis is on legal rights. While the decision of courts may well represent the values of our society, those values are not ipso facto morally binding for everyone. There is still the obligation of moral accountability from which the physician cannot be excused by a court decision.

This obligation becomes extremely important if the courts move in the direction of the most recent opinion of the Superior Court of California for the County of Los Angeles, in the *Bouvia* case dated April 16, 1986. In his concurring opinion, Judge Compton averred that the decision to withdraw a nasogastric tube was not only Bouvia's right, but that health professionals had an obligation to assist in Bouvia's intention to end her life.[18] The implications of such an opinion for individual physicians and for medical ethics are profound indeed. They extrapolate autonomy as an absolute principle, much as Engelhardt does in his book *The Foundations of Bioethics*.[19] Without rebutting Judge Compton or Engelhardt in detail here, we would say that these opinions illustrate why we feel that the restitution of beneficence is so important to medical ethics.

The *Bouvia* decision, in a sense, is proof of the opinions of one legal scholar that "the dynamics of court intervention merely confuse the lines of responsibility instead of clarifying them."[20] Burt argues that physicians should not take cases to court: "Physicians must be willing to assume some significant risk of adverse results, if only to force them to empathize with the patient who is also in the midst of a dilemma."[21] One may agree with Burt about the artificiality of court resolution of medical issues. But he seems insensitive to the loss of time, dignity, and reputation, and the mental anguish of court processes, as well as the overwhelming magnitude of cash awards juries are handing down these days. Nor is the likelihood of a suit an optimal, or even effective, way to "force" physicians to "empathize."

Burt's admonitions would have some moral force if the physician invokes the court simply to "immunize" himself or herself against suit. But the physician's use of the court to prevent moral harm in the interests of his patient is justified. Again, we must emphasize that the court decision does not resolve the substantive moral issue. Indeed, as in the *Bouvia* case or the case of *Roe v. Wade,* the court decision may be morally offensive.

In this view the courts should be used sparingly and in the interests of the patient. Under certain circumstances they may be the last resort for protecting the lives of those who cannot make their own decisions. This is particularly the case with never-competent infants, the retarded, or the psychotic, whose values and wishes cannot be known to others.

THE SPECIAL CASE OF INFANTS, THE RETARDED, AND THE PSYCHOTIC

With the never-competent patient the physician and family share guardianship for the welfare of the patient. We know, as occurred in the cases of *Baby Doe*[22] and *Baby Jane Doe,*[23] that parents and physicians may differ on the moral issue. The relative importance of family, physicians, and courts in decision making for infants, and the degree to which government regulations may intervene, have been the source of great controversy in the last several years.

The heated debates that surrounded the recommendations of the Department of Health and Human Services respecting the care of seriously ill and defective infants centered on the conflicting responsibilities of government, the family, and the medical profession.[24] The Department of Health and Human Services has argued that the state has an interest in the care of these infants, who should not be discriminated against because of their disabilities. The department's regulations and recommendations have undergone serial emendations. In their final form they recommend that terminally ill infants should be treated unless treatment is futile and excessively burdensome. Medications, food, and hydration are considered part of the mandatory care of such infants.

Professional associations, such as the American Academy of Pediatrics and the American College of Obstetrics and Gynecology, have objected on the grounds of protecting the right of privacy; they have asserted that the decision to withdraw or withhold treatment is a matter to be decided by parents and physicians and not by the courts or legislation.

In our view this amounts to granting parents absolute rights over the lives of their infants. While we affirm the view that the courts are not the place to settle ethical disputes, that they should be used sparingly, and that legislation concerning clinical decisions should be kept to a minimum, we do not agree that the state has no interest in protecting the lives of incompetent patients. Moreover, on the principle we have been enunciating in this book—beneficence-in-trust—we do not believe that the absolutization of parental autonomy is morally defensible. Indeed, the criteria for cessation of treatment delineated by the Department of Health and Human Services seem to us to provide the balance between autonomy and beneficence that we are convinced is necessary in the care of all patients, particularly the most vulnerable members of our society— infants, the retarded, and the psychotic. What is problematic, however, is the seemingly mandatory use of "appropriate" medications, fluids, and nutrition. Much depends as the definition of "appropriate." We hold that some treatments can, at times, be a burden and needlessly prolong dying.

Incompetent patients are precisely those most at risk in a society increasingly driven by utilitarian, economic, and libertarian impulses. Parents, by virtue of their bonding, ought to be the best advocates for infants or the retarded. But we also know that the undeniable realities and hardships involved in caring for the disabled and retarded can lead to unjustified decisions to undertreat. Physicians and other health workers have moral responsibilties for involving parents in decisions. They should abide by their decisions within the limits set by good moral practice. Best interests of a retarded or disabled infant are difficult to define, difficult enough that no group—parents, physicians, courts, governments—can be given the absolute right of determining those interests. Sustained dialogue, sharing of the moral obligation, and careful weighing of values in each case are essential to morally defensible decisions. Some tension between the parties is unavoidable and, indeed, may be necessary to protect the most vulnerable members of our society.

While we have not touched on the topic of social beneficence, it is important to add at this point that society is obligated to provide the necessary support services to make it possible to implement the decision to heal those who may not be fully functioning or self-supporting in later life. It is just this group of patients whose lives can be so easily and subtly disvalued on principles of utilitarianism or social benefit.

14

The Physician as Gatekeeper

An ethically perilous line of reasoning is gaining wide currency in our country today. It starts with a legitimate concern for rising health care costs, finds them uncontrollable by any means except some form of rationing, and concludes that the physician must become the "gatekeeper," the designated guardian of society's resources. Through both negative and positive financial incentives, it is reasoned, the physician can be forced to conserve tests, treatments, operations, hospitalizations, and referrals for consultation. In this way, supposedly, costs will be cut by eliminating "unnecessary" medical care.

From an economic point of view, this argument is attractive to those who must shoulder a good part of our more-than-a-billion-dollars-a-day health care bill. Policymakers, corporation executives, insurance carriers, affluent patients, and some physicians have already accepted the economic inevitability of rationing. The ethical implications are brushed aside as secondary, given the size of the problem and the fact that it is, indeed, physicians who are responsible for 75 percent of all health care expenditures.

Before committing ourselves to a course of action that will drastically alter the already strained trust between patients and physicians, some of the ethical questions associated with gatekeeping need closer examination.

To what extent can, or should, the physician serve simultaneously his or her own needs, the needs of patients, and those of society? To what extent should the physician be a double, triple, or even quadruple agent? Under what conditions would such divided advocacy be necessary, desirable, or morally licit?

What are the implications for our traditional understanding of medical ethics? How is the physician to resolve the conflicts of obligations built into divided advocacies? What is society's responsibility for creating or ameliorating these conflicts? Are these legal issues as well?

We argue that the line of reasoning that leads to rationing and physician gatekeeping is morally unsound and factually suspect; that there are conditions under which rationing might be morally justifiable, which are not met by current plans; and that we ought to minimize, rather than enhance, physician self-interest as a motive in medical and health care provision. We are well aware that this position resists the current popularity of justice and access discussions, which assume that rationing is a foregone conclusion and assign new roles to physicians.

We start with an examination of the conflict of interest that is a de facto aspect of physician-patient relationships. We then define three kinds of gate-keeping roles, the moral issues inherent in each, and the conditions for a morally licit rationing system.

DE FACTO CONFLICT OF INTEREST

When the first physician requested a fee for his services, economics and conflict of interest entered medicine.[1] Ever since, the physician's fee and the degree to which he could point to the necessity for his services to justify maintaining his own income have been sources of suspicion and contention between physicians and patients. Socrates, in his dialogue with the cynical Thrasymachus, was forced to admit that the physician was engaged in two "arts"—the art of medicine, which had as its end the health of the patient, and the art of making money, which had the physician's self-interest as its end and did not, in itself, contribute to the patient's welfare at all.

> Then isn't it the case that the doctor insofar as he is the doctor considers or commands not the doctor's advantage but that of the sick man? For the doctor in the precise sense was agreed to be a ruler of bodies and not a money maker.[2]
>
> Do you call the medical art the wage earner's art even if a man practicing medicine should earn wages?[3]
>
> The medical art produces health, the wage earner's art wages.[4]

Plato admitted through the voice of Socrates that these two arts could be in conflict, indeed had to be, given their disparate ends. For a more modern version of the fee dilemma, no one has more tellingly exposed the inevitability of a certain amount of conflict of interest in the physician's work than Shaw.[5]

This de facto conflict of interest is difficult or impossible to eliminate, given that physicians must earn a living, support families, and have access to the same material goods as others. What mitigates the conflict is the ethical commitment of the physician to the patient's good, that is, to the principle of beneficence.

Beneficence has always implied some degree of effacement of the physician's self-interest in favor of the interest of the patient. For centuries, good physicians have treated patients who could not pay, have exposed themselves to contagion or physical harm in responding to the call of the sick, and have sacrificed their leisure and time with their own families—sometimes too liberally—all out of commitment to serve the good of the sick.

Indeed, it is this effacement of self-interest that distinguishes a true profession from a business or craft.[6] And it is the expectation that physicians will, by and large, practice some degree of self-effacement that warrants the trust that society and individual patients place in them. It is the physician's public commitment to service beyond self-interest that constitutes the real entry of the medical graduate into the profession. The awarding of a medical degree signifies only successful completion of a course of study, but the oath is a public act of commitment to a special way of life demanded by the nature of medicine and the specific obligations that bind those who enter it.[7]

Ethical commitments can, and do, mitigate the conflicts of interest inherent in medical practice, but they do not eliminate them—except perhaps in the heroic examples of self-sacrifice we expect only of saints and martyrs. Surely, the salaried physician is not free of this impediment. If his financial incentives are reduced, other motives, including prestige, power, professional advancement, self-indulgence, unionization, and family obligations, can conflict with the care owed the patient. These can be just as detrimental to the patient's well-being as can the physician's monetary interests.

While there has always been some irreducible quantum of self-interest in medicine, rarely, if ever, has self-interest been socially sanctioned, morally legitimated, or encouraged as it is in the rationing approach to cost containment. Today the physician's self-interest is deliberately used by policymakers to contain the availability, accessibility, and quality of services to the patient. It is against this background of how they accentuate the de facto conflict of interest in medicine that the several forms of gatekeeping, licit and illicit, must be examined.

THREE FORMS OF GATEKEEPING

De Facto Gatekeeping: The Traditional Role

As with de facto conflict of interest, there is in the nature of the medical transaction an unavoidable gatekeeping function that the physician has always exercised and, indeed, is under compulsion to exercise in a morally defensible way. The unavoidable fact is that the physician recommends that tests, treatments, medications, operations, consultations, periods of stay in hospitals and nursing homes, and so forth meet the patient's needs.

This fact imposes a serious positive moral obligation on the physician to use both the individual's and society's resources optimally. In the case of the individual patient, the physician is obligated by his or her promise to act for the patient's welfare to use only those measures appropriate to cure the patient or alleviate his or her suffering. What the physician recommends must be *effective,* that is, it must materially modify the natural history of the disease, and it must also be *beneficial,* that is, it must be to the patient's benefit. Some measures— such as treatments for pneumonia—are highly effective, but may not be always beneficial if they unnecessarily prolong the act of dying and thus impose the burden of futility and expense without benefit for the patient. Other treatments benefit the patient but are not effective in altering the course of the disease—pain relief, nursing or home care, or intravenous fluids and nutrition.

The same distinction applies to diagnostic procedures. The physician has a moral obligation to use laboratory tests, X rays, and imaging procedures only if they contribute materially to the certitude of the diagnosis or the nature of the clinical decision. Marginally helpful tests, especially if they are expensive, or tests that are simply for teaching purposes (if the patient is in a teaching hospital) are not justifiable.

The physician, therefore, has a legitimate, indeed, a morally binding, responsibility to function as a gatekeeper. He must use his knowledge to practice competent, scientifically rational medicine. His guidelines should be diagnostic elegance (just the right degree of economy of means in diagnosis) and therapeutic parsimony (just those treatments that are demonstrably beneficial and effective). In this way the physician automatically fulfills several moral obligations: He avoids unnecessary risk to the patient from dubious treatment and he conserves the financial resources of both the patient and society.

The physician remains the patient's advocate. As the de facto gatekeeper, the physician is obliged to obtain tests and use treatments that are beneficial to his patient and not to restrict access for purely financial or economic reasons. The physician may withhold treatment if the patient decides that he does not wish to consume his family's resources. Thus, limiting access can be part of a legitimate gatekeeper role.

The role of de facto gatekeeper, when ethically performed, entails no conflict with the patient's good. Economics and ethics, individual and social good, and the doctor's and the patient's interests are all in congruence. In rational medicine, as we have defined it, the mode of the payment—whether by salary or fee—should make no difference. Properly conceived and practiced, rational medicine in a sense solves the dilemma posed in the first book of Plato's *Republic.* It subjects both the physician's art as physician and his art as wage earner to a higher standard—the standard of rational medicine that, in turn, derives its justification from the fact that is is in the patient's best interests. In the morally defensible gatekeeper role, the physician uses his de facto position to advance the good of his patient. In contrast, two new versions of gatekeeping have been introduced, each with attendant serious moral objection because their primary intent is economic, not ethical, obligation.

The Negative Gatekeeper Role

In the negative version of the gatekeeper role, the physician is placed under the constraints of self-interest to restrict the use of medical services of all kinds, but particularly those that are most expensive. A variety of measures is used, each of which interjects economic considerations into the physician's clinical decisions and limits his discretionary latitude in making decisions.

One way to do this is through the diagnostic-related group (DRG) program, which assigns in advance to more than four hundred disease categories a fixed sum or a fixed number of days of hospitalization. If the number of days (or tests, procedures, and so forth) is exceeded, the institution or the physician loses the difference; if the number of days of hospitalization is less than the standard allotment, then the institution or physician makes a profit.

In other plans the physician or institution contracts to provide care for some prescribed number of patients for a fixed annual sum. This can be an HMO or a preferred provider organization. Again, if the total costs for care exceed the contracted amount, the provider bears the loss; if the costs are less, the provider makes a profit. Variations on these themes are several, and they need not be detailed here. The essence of each is to motivate the provider to limit access to care by appealing to his or her self-interest.[8]

With all these plans the physician becomes the focus of incentives and disincentives in several ways: as a private practitioner when she hospitalizes a patient under the DRG system, and as the employee or partner in a prepayment insurance plan, such as an HMO, independent practice association, or primary care network. Increasingly, in each case, the physician's economic efficiency is monitored, and her deviations from the norm are rewarded or punished. The rewards may be in the form of profit sharing, bonuses, promotion in the organization, or other perquisites and preferments. The discentives are loss of profit, limits on admitting privileges, or nonrenewal of a coemployment contract. In some instances productivity and efficiency schedules, and other quantitative measures, not only of cost containment but of profit making, are used to evaluate the physician's performance.

The major pressure in these plans at present is upon the primary care physician, the first contact within of the health care system who makes the majority of decisions about entry into the system. The primary care physician may be the family primary practitioner, general internist, or pediatrician. The primary physician, as the "person in the trenches," has the greatest influence over access to expensive resources of hospitalization, testing, and consulting. For this reason, many prepayment plans insist that the patient stay with one primary care physician within the system, lest they shop around for one who might be more compliant. Gradually, as pressures for cost containment increase, the consultant and tertiary care specialists will very likely also be included as gatekeepers, with constraints and criteria suited to the nature of their specialties.

Positive Gatekeeping

The positive version of gatekeeping is less well defined and not usually explicitly formalized. In this version the physician is constrained to increase rather than decrease access to services. The purpose here is not containing costs but enhancing profits. For those who can pay, the latest and most expensive diagnostic or therapeutic services are offered; services are provided based on market "demand" rather than medical need. The aim is to "penetrate" or "dominate" the market to eliminate services that are not profitable. Increasing the demand for services is an implicit goal. Here the physician becomes virtually a salesperson. Already, we see this most blatantly in television and newspaper advertisements soliciting clients for elective surgery and all sorts of other services, some authentic and some quite useless.

With the positive gatekeeping role, the physician uses his or her de facto position as gatekeeper to his own financial advantage or to that of his employer. He shares in the profit directly if he is an owner of, or investor in, the service provided; he is rewarded by pay increases, advancement, and so on if he is employed.

THE MORAL ISSUES IN MEDICAL GATEKEEPING

Moral Issues in Negative Gatekeeping

Both the positive and negative versions of gatekeeping exploit the de facto position of the physician as the filter through which patients gain access to services. The purposes to be served, however, are not primarily in the patient's interests. The moral issues arise from the degree to which these other interests dilute the trust the patient places in the physician as his or her primary agent advocate. The motives of self-interest upon which the newer gatekeeping roles depend complicate and accentuate the irreducible quanta of self-interest that have always existed in the physician-patient relationship.

Efforts at cost containment are not, in themselves, immoral and, as noted above, are morally mandatory when they are in the best interests of the patient. They violate those interests if, for whatever reason, they deny needed services or induce the patient to demand, or the physician to provide, unneeded services. The ethical dilemmas of gatekeeping therefore arise out of the way economic incentives and disincentives modify the physician's freedom to act in the patient's behalf. While in the past the physician was largely responsible for defining necessary and unnecessary care, those determinations are now formularized by policy. In applying the formulae the physician becomes the agent of the hospital or the system, rather than the patient. And her medical criteria of necessary treatment are subject to modification or veto by economic considerations.

Many of these ethical dilemmas are illustrated in the Medicare prospective payment system now in force in the majority of states. In this system the cost-based per diem reimbursement system of the past is replaced by a prospective payment system based on fixed prices for 471 DRGs. The initial motivation behind this transition was to improve quality of care by linking it directly to reimbursement. Thus, it was reasoned that the DRG system would cut costs by closer scrutiny of care, aimed especially at limiting "unnecessary" tests, drugs, procedures, and hospitalization. Besides being economically wasteful, unneeded care is sometimes dangerous to patients.

These cost-containment measures are not intrinsically immoral. Certainly, we cannot consider them unethical simply because they limit the physician's latitude in decision making. Rather, it is the effect of this limitation on the patient that is ethically crucial, as is the moral responsibility of the physician operating within such a system when she deems its impact to be harmful for her patient.

The difficulty in the application of present DRG policies arises in the determination of what is "necessary" for quality care for a particular patient. In a system based on average lengths of stay for each disease, individual patients may suffer, since no two diseases manifest themselves in the same way in every patient. As a result, disease entities, not individual patients, are treated, and the original aim of quality care is compromised. Sometimes this is dangerous to patients who may be transferred or "dumped" as their reimbursement runs out.[9]

Further, the needs for hospitalization, tests, and medical care for a previously healthy, middle-aged head of a household with a comfortable home and a good job who is diagnosed as having pneumonia are very different from the needs of a chronically ill, elderly widow, living alone and far from her family, who has the same disease. Given the variable nature of patient responses to illness, a certain number of individual cases must fall outside the statistical projections. These are termed *outliers*—those who need lengthier stays, more procedures, more medications, and so on than the DRG plan allows.

Two tendencies that are deleterious to patients are already manifested in the way the DRG system is being administered in many hospitals. One is the fact that patients are being discharged "quicker and sicker." The second is the failure to provide the extra funds needed by the outlier. In both instances it is often the frail, elderly patient who is sent "home" with no adequate provision for posthospital care in a nursing home, at home, or elsewhere. (The American Association of Retired Persons has a hot line to call in case the elderly think they have been discharged too early.[10]) In fact, the trend in public policy at the moment is to curtail payment for nonhospital and long-term care, further aggravating the harm caused by premature discharge. This system is also reported to endanger the poor.[11]

In prospective payment systems the physician is automatically a negative gatekeeper. To the extent that unnecessary care is avoided and the quality of care receives closer scrutiny, the good of the patient is served. But when the system harms the patient, the question of the physician's primary agency arises. If she is primarily the patient's advocate, agent, and minister, she must protect the patient's interest against the system, even at the cost of some risk and damage to her own self-interest.

In addition to the intrinsic difficulties of gatekeeping, the physician's judgments are beclouded by a variety of pressures and motives inimical to the patient's interests.[12] There is, first of all, the tendency to underutilization since this rewards the physician or hospital. The temptation, therefore, is great to cut corners, to declare as "frills" what might otherwise be necessities, or to be less sensitive to the more subtle, but equally important, needs of patients for psychosocial support. A study of British physicians showed that, because of social pressure, what were once considered medically indicated treatments are now deemed unnecessary and not in the patient's best interests. All that has changed is the determination to ration.[13] Further, the primary care physician is encouraged to temporize in her workup and to delay expensive tests, treatments, or consultations. This is especially the case in HMOs. The physician may even stretch her competence dangerously to do certain procedures herself in order to contain costs.

Another pressure in prospective payment plans is to disfavor or disenfranchise the sicker patients, those with chronic illnesses and those who need more expensive care. A study of Rush St. Luke's Hospital in Chicago demonstrated that the elderly in the intensive care unit will have to receive a much lower quality of care because the DRG system pays the hospital an average of twelve thousand dollars per patient less than it costs to treat them.[14] Less admirable still is the way cost containment can be used, consciously and unconsciously, to justify the exclusion or denial of services to difficult, troublesome, or obnoxious patients, or to other categories of patients one prefers not to see—the neurotic, the "complainers," the "hypochondriacs"—or, worst of all, the ethnic or social groups one dislikes personally.

Another deleterious effect of negative gatekeeping is to cultivate competition among providers on the wrong grounds. Instead of competition to provide the highest-quality care, as judged by the standards of rational medicine, there is competition for the best records of savings, productivity, and efficiency, the shortest hospital stays, or the least number of procedures done. Granted that excesses of care exist and are deleterious, it still does not follow that underutilization is beneficial, especially with certain very effective though costly high-technology procedures (for example, renal dialysis, organ transplant, coronary angioplasty, CAT scanning, and nuclear magnetic resonance examinations).

To be effective, many prospective payment plans insist that patients be locked into receiving care from one primary care physician. The choice of physicians and the freedom to switch is severely limited. The most sensitive part of the healing relationship, the confidence one must have in one's personal physician, is thus ignored or compromised. Especially in chronic or recurrent disease, this confidence is essential to effective care.

These factors converge to drive the physician's self-interest into conflict with the patient's. These conflicts are heightened by the rather drastic changes occurring in the economic status of the medical professional, which make the physician more vulnerable to economic pressure. Currently, there is an oversupply of physicians in urban areas and in many specialties.[15] Many physicians now graduate with debts for their education in the neighborhood of one hundred thousand dollars. The high cost of malpractice premiums must be laid out before anyone dares risk even a day of medical practice. Competition from corporately owned and operated clinics forces even conscientious physicians into "survival" tactics of questionable moral defensibility.

The result of all this is that many young, and even older, physicians are driven into salaried group practices and automatically become negative gate-keepers. The physician's independence, as Starr has shown, is rapidly eroding, and with it her ability to withstand the institutional and corporate strictures on her judgment about what is good for her patient.[16] It is becoming ever more costly, personally and financially, for even the most morally sensitive physician to practice the effacement of self-interest that beneficence-in-trust requires.

Moral Issues in Positive Gatekeeping

The moral conflicts in the positive version of gatekeeping are less subtle. Here the profit motive is primary. The transaction between physician and patient becomes a commodity transaction. The physician becomes an independent entrepreneur or the hired agent of entrepreneurs and investors who themselves have no connection with the traditions of medical ethics. The physician begins to practice the ethics of the marketplace, to think of his or her relationship with the patient not as a covenant or trust, but as a business and a contract relation-ship. Ethics becomes not a matter of obligations or virtue, but of legality. The metaphors of business and law replace those of ethics. Medical knowledge becomes proprietary, the doctor's private property to be sold to whom he chooses at whatever price and condition he chooses.

When positive gatekeeping is employed, the dependence, anxiety, lack of knowledge, and vulnerability of the sick person (or even the healthy person) are exploited for personal profit. To encourage unnecessary cosmetic surgery, hys-terectomies, CAT scans, or sonograms, even if the patient believes he or she ought to have "the latest and the best," is to defect from even the most primor-dial concept of stewardship of the patient's interest. Here the conflict of interest is more blatant than in the negative version of gatekeeping. The patient becomes primarily a source of income. The more crass financial motives that have moti-vated selfish physicians are legitimated and even given social sanction.

In the positive version of gatekeeping, there is not, as there may be in the negative version, any defensible moral argument. Some defend the profit motive as necessary to medical progress, to maintain quality of service or even to pro-vide charitable care. It would be unrealistic to deny that for some physicians these are the only effective motives and that some good can come of them. But, ultimately, when a conflict occurs between profit and patient welfare, patient welfare is sure to suffer. The unrestrained monetary instinct corrupts medicine as surely as do unrestrained instincts for power or prestige.

SOME SOCIAL-ETHICAL CONCOMITANTS OF RATIONING

The negative and positive gatekeeping roles both involve social consequences of dubious moral probity. Both tolerate and, indeed, foster two or more levels of quality, availability, and accessibility of health care. The affluent person can buy whatever he or she needs or wants; he can supplement what a DRG plan allows if he is an outlier. The various prepayment plans and organizations eagerly seek to enroll him. The less affluent and the poor have no such access to care. They may or may not be assured of what is called an "adequate" level of care. Adequacy is vaguely defined, but on close examination it will be inevitable that the differences between what rich and poor receive will be significant. The poor and the lower economic strata of the middle class are relegated to public hospitals, which will have to be reestablished and, of course, financed.

The difference in the care provided in public and "private" hospitals extends beyond convenience, accommodations, or "frills," Anyone whose experience goes back to the large municipal hospitals of several decades ago will recognize these differences. The efforts of the last two decades to undo the injustices of a multilevel system of health care are being reversed by the move to rationing, cost containment, and gatekeeping.

A different kind of social-ethical issue arises if we ask whether it is defensible for society to transpose its responsibility for rationing to the physician. Are not the criteria for these decisions the responsibility of all of us? In situations of extreme economic exigency, rationing could be justified. But the criteria for rationing and the principle of justice to be followed should rest with society, not with the physician. There is no assurance that the physician is any more fair or just than others in deciding who shall receive so crucially important a resource as health care. Do we as a society really want to give this kind of power to physicians?

It is necessary to strike a very careful balance between societally determined criteria for rationing and the latitude allowed physicians in making rationing decisions. Society may wish to use the DRG mechanism as a way of expressing its value choices, but should the physician accept such a charge in the face of his or her prime duty to be the patient's advocate?

On grounds of the conflict it generates between physician and patient interests and the social injustice it fosters, the role of gatekeeper entails an erosion and a violation of the commitment to patient welfare that must be the primary moral imperative in medical care. This commitment flows from the nature of illness and the promise to service made by individual physicians and the profession as a whole. That commitment has a basis in the empirical nature of the healing relationship, in which a sick person—dependent vulnerable, exploitable—must seek out the help of another who has the necessary knowledge, skill, and facilities to effect a cure. It is inevitably a relationship of unequal freedom and power, in which the stronger party is obligated to protect the interest of the weaker.[17]

SOME COUNTERARGUMENTS

Some would argue that the moral issues we have raised against gatekeeping, rationing, and for-profit medicine on grounds of conflicts of interest and divided loyalties are specious. The opposing viewpoints are several: Medical care has always been rationed (tragic choices have always been made in which some do not receive adequate care);[18] differences in availability, accessibility, and quality have always existed and always will; even the so-called not-for-profit hospitals make an "excess" of revenues over expenditures. Moreover, the doctor's fee is itself a "profit" and a source of conflict of interest. And even if this were not true, rationing and fiscal motivations are essential to fiscal survival. Even religiously sponsored institutions argue that they must make a profit and must ration care according to the ability to pay. "No margin, no mission," they say. Survival, it is argued, demands practices that may be distasteful and unfair but not unjust.

We respond to these arguments as follows: First of all, the existence of inequity and injustice does not give them any necessary moral sanction, nor does the fact that all injustice cannot be eliminated in an imperfect world. If we cannot afford all the health care people want or need, we can find other ways of rationing or allocating resources that are more morally valid than those now in use. While tragic choices must always be made, they can be made on the basis of a more thoroughly thought-out national plan.

Second, there is a real difference between the way a for-profit and a not-for-profit institution handles the "excess" of revenue over expenditures. In a for-profit (more decorously called "investor-owned") hospital, the primary aim is profit because the prime obligation is to protect and enlarge the investor's shares. This, it must be added, is a moral obligation since the for-profit hospital is the steward of other people's money. The "profit," however, goes into the pockets of the investors, while in a not-for-profit hospital most of it must go into improvement of patient care services, capital expansion, and so forth. When the physician is a gatekeeper in a for-profit hospital, he or she has conflicting obligations—to the investor and to the patient.

Proponents of rationing point to the overutilization of services, inefficiency of management and operation, and lack of stimulus for innovative models of care that admittedly beset cost-reimbursement and government entitlement programs. We cannot defend these shortcomings or argue for a "blank check" approach to health care. Both must be eliminated in any defensible system of health care payment. But the fact is that the various cost-containment systems now being used have yet to achieve greater efficiency than not-for-profit systems.[19] Indeed, it appears that in the for-profit system, gatekeeping has resulted in no cost advantage over not-for-profit systems, while the charges are higher (sometimes by as much as 25 percent). Thus, successful cost containment, the major moral justification for gatekeeping, is questionable since prices are not appreciably lower. Yet, today, few people have adequate insurance coverage, and more are forced to deplete their financial reserves to pay for needed medical care.

Some would argue that we have in the professional standards review organization mechanism all the controls we need to prevent abuses of the prepayment systems. These organizations were established in every state to monitor the quality of cost of services provided under Medicare. They are peer review organizations composed of physicians whose function is to assure quality of care and containment of costs by avoidance of unnecessary procedures. Because of concerns about the efficiency and assiduity of their policing of physician performance, they were reorganized by Congress in 1985. Since then, the number of disciplinary actions has increased notably.

It is an essential moral duty of physicians as individuals and as members of these review organizations to monitor, correct, and discipline abuses by doctors and hospitals. The organizations should obviously be employed as effectively as possible, but they do not solve the ethical dilemmas of gatekeeping. What they should assure is that the de facto gatekeeping functions are carried out and rational and honest medicine is practiced.[20] Professional standards review organizations cannot eradicate the dilemmas created for the conscientious doctor by a national policy of rationing in which he must function as a gatekeeper.

For the dishonest or incompetent physician, the ethical dilemmas are inconsequential. It is the physician committed to the good of his patient, the one who practices rational medicine, for whom divided loyalties are a genuine ethical problem. For such a physician, even the professional standards review organization might pose an ethical dilemma—for example, when peer reviewers censure him for failing to apply cost-containment measures if he sincerely believes failing to do so will serve his patient. Effective peer review mechanisms are essential to good care. It is the ethical implications of the health policies under which they operate that must be subjected to critical scrutiny.

IS RATIONING INEVITABLE?

The only argument for rationing that has some moral substance is economic necessity. Some fear that rising health care costs will seriously compromise availability and accessibility of other good things our society needs to thrive, such as food, housing, jobs, and national security. This is the justification for efforts to put some arbitrary ceiling on the percentage of gross national product dedicated to health care. Is the assumption of national bankruptcy by health care costs correct? If it is, rationing might be justified. Then the moral question becomes, under what conditions? If it is not, then rationing has no moral sanction.

The question turns on the validity of the initial premise that leads to inevitable rationing. This is a difficult question to answer because comparable figures on national expenditures for other things we as a society want are hard to come by. Moreover, whether or not there is a crisis depends very much on the value we place on other expenditures. Some of the data on health care costs that policymakers find distressing are presented below.

The U.S. total health care bill has now exceeded 1 billion dollars per day. The percentage of our gross national product allotted to health care is higher than almost any other nation's and is rising each year. About 2.5 billion dollars is spent on keeping 85,000 patients with chronic renal disease alive.[21] Approximately 4.4 billion dollars is spent for heart and liver transplants. Ten percent of all operating costs of a university hospital goes into the last three to six months of life. Eighty percent of those who die do so in a hospital, as compared with 50 percent in 1949 and a much smaller percentage at the turn of the century. Almost 230,000 babies are born each year weighing less than 2,500 grams. Of the half who survive, 15 percent end up with some residual defect. Two billion dollars is spent each year on neonatal intensive care units.

Each of these and other figures have been selected as the place to economize by some proponent of rationing. Rationing for these groups is proposed on utilitarian, economic, and humanitarian grounds—that is, to reduce the number of dependent, nonproductive members of society, or to save money for other socially useful purposes or needs, or to prevent dooming the retarded and the disabled to lives of poor "quality." Some suggest that persons over a certain age should not be offered dialysis (a policy followed in England for persons older than 55 years); that high-technology procedures such as liver and heart transplants or even coronary bypass surgery should not be performed; that research in high-technology treatments such as artificial hearts be halted; that babies under a certain cutoff weight should not be treated; that there should be a monetary limit on the expenditures for persons with terminal illnesses in the last few months of life; or that those above a certain age should not be treated vigorously.

These proposals deserve more critical examination than is possible here. They illustrate a range of policy options, all of which center on rationing of expensive forms of care. Against these expenditures we must consider expenditures for the following that, as a nation, we make willingly, indeed, sometimes avidly: 40 billion dollars for alcohol, 30 billion for tobacco, 65 billion for cosmetics, 65 billion for advertising, and unspecified billions for recreational handguns, illicit drugs, gambling, and various types of luxuries.[22]

What decision would we make if we consciously compared these expenditures with those for health care? Is 2.5 billion dollars too much to spend on keeping seventy thousand people with renal disease alive—many of them living active lives—or a projected 4 billion dollars to return thousands of people to active lives by means of cardiac, liver, or renal transplants, which are becoming more effective each year? What about the 50 percent of underweight babies who *do* survive and the 85 percent of those who are not disabled or retarded? Can we decide what is a "quality" life for another person, especially for an infant whose values cannot possibly be known? How do we distinguish between futile and burdensome treatments and effective, though expensive, lifesaving treatments? How do we protect the vulnerable—the old, the very young, the poor, and the socially outcast—from being discriminated against in rationing decisions? How do we know when research into high technology may turn out to be beneficial for all, rather than for a few?

How would we answer these questions if we considered health of higher value than some of the other things for which we make great expenditures without question? Would we have to ask these questions at all if we could cut out truly unnecessary care, reduce inefficiencies of the care we now give, and establish some priority among the categories of care based on their need, benefit, and effectiveness as seen from the patient's point of view?

If we address these questions in an orderly way, identifying the underlying values and making conscious choices, we might decide that rationing and lifeboat ethics are not warranted in this country today. It would take more space than this chapter permits to establish these contentions. The questions have yet to be examined carefully, particularly to expose their underlying value desiderata. This is a sensitive operation, and one whose conclusions might prove embarrassing. How we make the choices rationing implies will reveal more about the kind of people we are, and wish to be, than it would about the ideals we profess.

THE CONDITIONS FOR MORALLY LICIT RATIONING

Let us assume that there is a true economic crisis, that health needs are, indeed, eroding society's capacity to obtain other needed goods—housing, jobs, food, security—and that we have consciously come to the conclusion that rationing and lifeboat ethics are necessary on moral grounds. Under these conditions we must face opposing moral obligations: to provide health care and at the same time protect the fabric of society. Such conditions exist in times of natural disaster, war, epidemics, and the like. Under these conditions rationing of health and many other things is accepted. But even under less urgent conditions, morally valid criteria can be established for both allocation and rationing of national resources dedicated to health and medical care. A tentative set of criteria is described below.

First of all, all alternatives to rationing should have been exhausted. We are far from such a goal. To attain it, we would have to assure at least the following:

1. The efficiency of management of personnel, facilities, and fiscal resources must be optimal. This is not the place to detail how the necessary measures are to be employed. Suffice it to say that economies have been and can still be made in this area. They must be made first if rationing is to be justified as a national policy.

2. Rational medicine, defined above as consisting of diagnostic elegance and therapeutic parsimony, would have to be practiced universally and optimally. The elimination of unnecessary tests would save in the range of 15 to 20 billion dollars per year. An even larger sum could be saved by the elimination of truly unnecessary surgery, medications, and other therapeutic procedures. A similar amount might be saved by transferring dying patients to hospice care, or by requiring advance directives of retiring persons soon to move into the Social Security system.[23] An estimate of the amount saved by these measures is difficult to obtain since much depends on the definition of "unnecessary."[24]

3. Some hierarchy of services would have to be established to govern the priority assigned to various kinds of health care expenditures. To be morally valid this hierarchy must be ordered from the patient's point of view according to benefit, effectiveness, and need. In one possible hierarchy, highly effective preventive measures for diseases of wide distribution—for example, immunization for smallpox, tetanus, diptheria, pertussis, polio—might come first. Genetic screening and manipulation would fall into this category as well. Then could follow beneficial and effective treatments for life-threatening disease—for example, emergency trauma care, renal dialysis, angioplasty in impending myocardial infarction, radiation and chemotherapy for responsive neoplastic disease, and

the like. The next category might be beneficial and effective treatment for less acute but serious disease—coronary bypass surgery for intractable angina pectoris, surgery for disabling hernia, and drug treatment for gout, peptic ulcer, and hypertension. Less urgent would be expenditures for expensive treatments with marginal benefit, such as coronary bypass when medical treatment is equally effective, carotid endarterectomy of certain types, preventive cholecystectomy for cholelithiasis, and so on. Next would be effective treatments for nondisabling, non–life-threatening disorders—for instance, purely cosmetic surgery. The expenditures of lowest priority would be those for experimental treatments such as transplant of fetal brain tissue into adult brains, artificial hearts, and other treatments whose testing at this stage yields only marginal benefits.

This list is obviously a subject for vigorous debate as to content and priority. Our point is not to argue for this particular ranking, but to suggest that establishing such a hierarchy is one precondition to morally licit rationing.

A similar hierarchical listing would have to be developed for diagnostic procedures as well. Many of these are expensive and add only marginally to diagnostic accuracy. With diagnosis, as with treatment, the latest is not always the best. The additional benefit or effectiveness may not be sufficient to warrant the added expense.

We must be reminded that many acceptable ways to manage patients do not necessarily involve the most sophisticated technologies. Some of these, indeed, may even be preferable since they may be less risky than the latest procedures. Tests done solely in the interests of "defensive medicine" to forestall litigation would have to be eliminated. Despite the physician's understandable fear of malpractice suits, he or she cannot morally justify the costs or risk of unnecessary procedures simply to protect himself or herself. Of course, this would realistically require a national cap on malpractice suit awards, something generally needed in the current insurance crisis.

Assuming that the above and other measures to contain costs have been utilized fully, the next condition for morally licit rationing is the open public discolsure of the categories of care that will be rationed, together with the principles upon which they will be rationed. Selection of a morally defensible rationing principle is another difficult but unavoidable condition of a morally defensible rationing system.

Shall the principle be equity of access for all, or age, social worth, merit, ability to pay, or lottery? Arguments have been marshalled to defend one or another principle of distributive justice. Again, we cannot examine each principle critically here.[25] We wish simply to establish the need of settling on some explicit principle. Once established, that principle must be made known to all. As it is, a variety of principles are in use and only rarely are explicitly stated. Again, the principle we select will tell much about our most cherished values, the kind of society we wish to be, and whether we regard health as a human right, a social obligation, or simply another commodity.

An especially crucial requirement with respect to the gatekeeper role is that the hierarchy of services and the principle of rationing be determined in public policy and made known to all who seek care. It is not to be left up to the physician to determine in individual cases who lives or dies, who gets care and who does not. In this way the physician can remain the primary advocate of the patient, albeit within constraints imposed by social or public policy established at a national level.

The physician may disagree with those constraints when he feels they are injurious to patients—his own or others. When he does so, he has a moral obligation to use the means available in a democratic society to change policies, regulations, or procedures that violate his perception of what is good for patients. He can function with moral integrity in the "valid" de facto gatekeeping role we have described above. In that role he serves his patient's interests, not his own or those of the institution or corporation providing health care services.

But the invalid roles of negative and positive gatekeeper, as defined in this chapter, require the physician to dilute his primary advocacy of his patient's interest. Society should not force or encourage physicians to be double or triple agents. It is not morally defensible for society to "unload" its unpleasant rationing decisions on physicians. Nor can it run the risk of physician bias or prejudice in the way resources are rationed in individual cases. Patients who are denied some needed care must recognize that it is the whole of society that has denied them, under constraints that apply to everyone. Physicians are free to protest unjust measures and to educate the public and policymakers to the dangers of their own rationing decisions. As a consequence the convenant of beneficence between physician and patient is preserved. The one who is ill need not fear that a physician is acting as a hidden double or triple agent. The physician, on his part, is under serious obligation to protect his patient's interest within the constraints imposed by health policies, but is also morally obligated to oppose and resist such policies when they prove injurious to his patients.

It is possible that our society will choose other things over health, that it will see health care as nothing more than a commodity or service like any other, and that it will impose the responsibility of specific rationing decisions on physicians. If this occurs it is a moral requirement that physicians publicly acknowledge the drastic difference this will make in the expectations the patient brings to his or her relationship with a doctor. The profession must signal the importance of the gatekeeper role in transforming medical ethics from a primary concern for individual patients to a competing concern for social or economic good. Were we to take this direction in medical ethics, we would be moving in the direction of the code of the Soviet physician, which makes the good of the polity and society the prime principle of medical ethics. Beneficence, patient autonomy, and justice—the cornerstones of professional medical ethics today—would have to yield to social good and economic need.

SOME LEGAL QUESTIONS

Neither the profession nor the public can have it both ways: Either the physician primarily serves the interests of the patient or the physician becomes the instrument of social and fiscal policy as well as patient good.

We cannot predict how the American people will ultimately resolve the serious ethical dilemmas of gatekeeping and whether they are prepared to accept the ethical conflicts of divided loyalty. There is, however, some indication that the public may not be ready to abandon its moral expectation that the physician act as the patient's primary agent. This is reflected in the potential for litigation in which patients hold physicians liable for harm done to them by premature discharge from the hospital, through the omission of tests, or failure to hospitalize under DRG and other cost-containment prepayment plans.

One distressing legal development is the possiblity that standards of care to which physicians are held will be downgraded to accommodate the kinds of decisions prospective payment will require. This possibility is already being discussed tentatively in the legal profession. The presumption is that standards can be lowered without loss of safety and that the public will accept "Chevrolet" in place of "Cadillac" care as long as it costs less.[26]

These assumptions are dangerous and invalid. They presume that lowering standards will mean simply eliminating "unnecessary" care or the "frills" and luxuries. Unfortunately, such distinctions are very hard to make since the differences between present and proposed standards are not all that trivial. It is very questionable whether such a move would decrease the possibility of suit or whether the doctor could be freed of his or her first duty to protect the patient. Moreover, there is very little likelihood that the American public would accept the implications of a lowered standard were it to be openly announced. When it comes to health care, very few people are willing to compromise their own safety.

Does the patient have a legal right to know in advance that a clinical decision has been made on economic rather that strictly medical grounds? Is the doctor to be held responsible for damage resulting from adherence to a national health care policy? Or is she liable if she does not violate such a policy when it has the potential to harm her patient? What penalty does she suffer for placing loyalty to a patient above loyalty to public or fiscal policy? Is it morally defensible for society to put the physician in the midst of such ethical and legal dilemmas?

Must informed consent in the future include full disclosure of the fact that economic or social criteria will be used to modify judgments made on scientific criteria or patient need? Will living wills have to take account of the fact and direct physicians to use economic criteria when deciding on starting and stopping life-support or other measures? These and other legal issues impinge upon and complicate the ethical dilemmas we have described in the two other gatekeeper roles now being assigned to physicians. Intensive examination of the legal issues and the provision of appropriate legal safeguards for both the patient and the physician must be devised if we, as a nation, go the route of rationing in toto, or even in part, as prepayment plans already in existence require.

This examination has already been precipitated by litigation surrounding one of the most common practices of prepayment and for-profit plans and institutions worried about deficits—the practice of "economic transfer."[27] When a patient presents for admission, his or her insurance coverage and ability to pay are assessed along with his or her medical condition. If the patient seems an economic risk, she is transferred to a public or religiously sponsored institution.

These transfers are made when the patient is presumed to be in a "stable" condition. However, the definition of stability varies considerably from physician to physician, and patients have suffered physical damage, to say nothing of emotional trauma, as a result.[28] It is a fact that the definition of a "stable state" is altered by economic considerations when a physician is an employee of an institution or a member of the resident staff.

The conflict of interest here is obvious and explicit. Clearly, the primary moral responsibility of the physician is to the patient. She puts herself at considerable risk—legal as well as moral—when she approves an economic transfer. Once again, we observe the paradox of an economic and market system exploiting the physician's self-interest and the public's expectation that the physician must act in the patient's best interests.

CONCLUSION

The physician is responsible for 75 percent of the nation's expenditures for health care. He or she is the gatekeeper who can limit or facilitate access to tests, treatments, consultations, and admission to a variety of health care institutions. There are three ways in which the physician can function as gatekeeper: one is morally mandatory, one is morally questionable, and one is morally indefensible.

The first is the traditional, or de facto, function, which imposes the responsibility to practice rational medicine—that is, to use only those diagnostic and therapeutic modalities that are beneficial and effective for the patient. This function rests on beneficence-in-trust. The proper exercise of traditional gatekeeping is not only morally imperative but economically sound.

The second form is negative gatekeeping usually within some form of prepayment system in which the physician strives to limit the use of health care services. This role is morally dubious because it generates a conflict between the responsibilities of the physician as a primary advocate of the patient and as guardian of society's resources. Under certain carefully defined conditions of economic necessity and moral monitoring, a negative gatekeeping role might be morally justifiable.

The third form is positive gatekeeping, in which the physician encourages the use of health care facilities and services for personal or corporate profit. This is an indefensible form of gatekeeping. No moral justification can be mustered in its favor.

Recognition of the ethical dilemmas created by the growing national belief that health care rationing is inevitable, and their impact on the care of patients and the ethics of the physician-patient relationship are matters of wide public concern. Significant legal issues are also emerging. As we have suggested here, the role of moral rationing is a true responsibility flowing from the principle of fiduciary beneficence. "No servant can serve two masters: for either he will hate the one, and love the other, or else he will hold to the one and despise the other. You cannot serve God and mammon."[29]

15

Beneficence-in-Trust:
How It Is Applied

Up to this point we have argued that promoting the patient's good requires restoration of beneficence to medical ethics in a way that takes into account, but does not capitulate to, autonomy. Our contention has been that the circumstances of clinical medicine ultimately require the patient to place his well-being in the care of the physician, and that this fact imposes on the physician a serious obligation of stewardship for the patient's best interests.

In this chapter we wish to illustrate how this principle operates in several concrete clinical situations. The central issue in clinical decisions will be: What is, in fact, in the patient's best interests? After all, few physicians would consciously act against what they believe to be their patient's good. Yet, the center of ethical debate is located at just that point—a sharp difference of opinion about what is a particular patient's good.

We believe that beneficence-in-trust provides a guideline—a principle of discernment, as it were—that points to a morally superior decision. We shall attempt to validate this assertion by examining a series of well-known court cases, some of them landmarks, in medical ethics. In each case we will try to show how our line of argument might modify the decision reached, or resolve some of the ethical dilemmas raised in these cases.

IN RE QUINLAN

Karen Ann Quinlan[1] was a young woman in a persistent vegetative state, possibly occasioned by drug overdosage. She had not appointed anyone as her legal guardian, nor had she made a living will. She had intimated that she would not want to live under certain conditions analogous to those in which she presented at the time of her hospital admission. Her parents and pastoral counselor agreed that a respirator should be withdrawn. Her physician disagreed. The case went to court, and what is now a landmark decision was handed down, establishing the right of parental surrogates to have a respirator withdrawn.

Quinlan's own wishes had been rather clear, and they were presented by the family in a credible way. There was no doubt that Quinlan would not have wanted her life prolonged on a respirator. As far as could be determined, she interpreted her good as discontinuance of life-support measures.

Quinlan's physician defined her good in another way: as preservation of her life by carrying out the medical indication—respiratory assistance. In our view the physician reduced the patient's good to one dimension—medical good—while ignoring the other levels of patient good we have defined and reversing the priority of good. In our scheme of the hierarchy of values, the patient's assessment of her own welfare, and her inherent dignity as a person to express her own values take precedence over medical good. Further, from the point of view of the process of decision making, the dialogical, consensual, fiduciary model of decision making was not used. We would conclude that, on both substance and procedure, the patient's best interests were not served by needlessly prolonging her life on a respirator.

In our view the physician's interpretation of beneficence was misguided. We would not deem it a responsible exercise of beneficence to continue life support when the prognosis is hopeless and nothing is achievable except the prolongation of death. Also, to violate the patient's wishes, provided they are not in conflict with some equally valid moral principle, is to violate her humanity and to use paternalism for harm rather than good.

The court's ruling placed the focus of decision on Quinlan's prognosis, and its locus in the hands of her family and physicians. Nonetheless, the recommendation of an ethics committee is problematic. If the patient's family meets the criteria for morally valid surrogate decisions and properly presents the patient's wishes based on her own values, and if the physician's dismal prognosis is well substantiated, there should be no need for further clarification or consultation as recommended by the court. In Quinlan's case much of the early debate centered on the reversibility of her condition. In such an instance a responsible physician would want to check his or her diagnosis and prognosis with others. Beneficence-in-trust would call for such consultation before discontinuance of life-support measures.

IN RE SAIKEWICZ

Joseph Saikewicz,[2] a retarded adult who had never been competent, contracted adult leukemia. The Belchertown State Home, in which he lived, wished to pursue treatment of his disease. Family members disagreed. The case went to the Massachusetts Supreme Court, which decided that Saikewicz should not be treated since he could not understand the course of the treatment. In effect, the court "substituted" its judgment for the patient's. The court also asserted that it should be involved in health care decisions (see chapter 13).

Reaction to this decision was swift and strong. Physicians and ethicists disagreed with the use of the standard of substituted judgment for a patient who had never been competent. Not only had Saikewicz not made his wishes known, his values and preferences could, by definition, never be known. Consequently, there could be no discussion of presumed wishes nor could a value history, as we have suggested, be employed (chapter 13). Thus, employing the substituted judgment doctrine seems a judicial sleight of hand. In this doctrine's strict form, one "substitutes," by presumption in the present, a judgment or decision based on how patients have made previous judgments.[3] This was not possible for Saikewicz. Instead, substituted judgment appeared to take the form of a quality-of-life judgment: "Mr. Saikewicz should not be treated because we, in his condition and with his degree of retardation, would not want to be treated."[4]

We would argue that in a never-competent patient like Saikewicz, whose values cannot be ascertained, the physician or other surrogates are reduced to a medical-indications standard. This does not imply treatment under all circumstances, but it does mean that treatments that are both effective and beneficial can be presumed to be in the patient's interest. This is not the same as a "reasonable person" standard since a reasonable person can introduce value desiderata not possible for someone like Saikewicz. Instead, the presumption ought to be that the patient should be treated if some benefit that outweighs harms and burdens can come of it.

In our view it would violate beneficence-in-trust to take quality of life, or the fact of mental retardation, into consideration. We cannot ascertain what the patient would consider a "quality existence." Nor can we discriminate against the patient because he is retarded and his quality of life is not acceptable to us.

Another problem in the Saikewicz case was the court's opinion that all such cases should be adjudicated by the courts. Physicians[5] and lawyers[6] took strong exception to this provision on logistic grounds and because of the distance of the court from the urgency and intimacy of the decision on the part of the patient's family and physician. In our view of the matter—if the criteria for morally valid surrogate decisions obtain—the patient's best interests are more likely to be served if the decision is made at the bedside, where the most intimate knowledge of the patient resides.

This is not to deny the obvious place of the court when there is no agreement at the bedside, when the criteria for morally valid surrogate decisions are lacking, or when some grievous harm or injustice is being done even though physician and family might agree. This was the case with Baby Doe, the "Bloomington Baby," an infant with Down's syndrome and an easily correctable defect who was allowed to starve to death. Concern about this decision moved beyond the judicial system and led to national and state legislation which sought to protect the retarded.[7]

NEJDL AND BARBER

Two California physicians, Drs. Neil Barber and Robert Nejdl,[8] were indicted for murder after withdrawing food and water from a patient who had suffered cardiac arrest after surgery and from whom the respirator had already been withdrawn. Withdrawals of treatment were done with the consent of the patient's wife. The case was brought to the attention of the district attorney's office by a nurse from the intensive care unit who, earlier during the patient's course, had refused to disconnect the respirator. The case was eventually decided on appeal in favor of the physicians.

Again, we would view the decision from the point of view of the guardianship of the patient's best interests by family and physician. The question is not whether administration of food and nutrition under these circumstances is treatment like any other.[9] Rather, beneficence dictates that we ascertain, to the best of our abilities, what serves some beneficial purpose in a patient who is in a permanent vegetative state. If certain procedures make the patient more comfortable and do not impose severe burdens, they ought to be continued.[10] Making the patient comfortable, easing pain, and caring for the patient's needs are always justifiable ends. Directly intending the death of the patient is not a form of beneficence that can be countenanced, though it has been advanced as a reason for direct euthanasia by libertarians.

Food and hydration can become so burdensome that their primary ends are frustrated—that is, benefiting the terminal patient by making him or her more comfortable. Surely, this is the case with a mentally competent patient who is terminal and refuses food because of anorexia or nausea, or even because she is prepared to die and sees no benefit in prolonging the act of dying. Such a patient can be allowed to take or refuse food or fluid as she wishes. The patient judges that the treatment provides no proportionate benefit.[11]

With a comatose patient in a permanent vegetative state, we cannot know for certain whether withholding food and fluids is causing discomfort.[12] Nor can we ascertain the degree to which noxious sensory signals are received by the damaged brain. Experienced clinicians know that comatose patients who recover sometimes startle them by what they "remember" about events that went on at the bedside when they were clinically unresponsive.

Beneficence dictates that we give the patient the benefit of any doubts. We can reason from the situation with mentally competent, terminally ill patients. In practice, they often refuse food while taking water and fluids, or at least seek to have their mouths and mucous membranes moistened. This suggests that, in terms of comfort, hydration may be more important than nutrition and, if not burdensome, ought to be continued.

When do hydration and nutrition become excessively burdensome? That is difficult to determine for a patient in a permanent vegetative state, in whom a nasogastric tube often must be repeatedly replaced, is persistently pulled out, or is accompanied by regurgitation of stomach contents into the lungs and a repeatedly leaking or infected gastrostomy. Fluids may become burdensome when peripheral or central portals of entry become difficult or inaccessible, and when imparied cardiovascular-renal function makes cardiac failure and pulmonary congestion a constant threat.[13]

It is not inappropriate to consider the unnecessary burden on medical attendants and staff of forcibly placing and maintaining artificial means of nutrition and hydration when there is no benefit to be gained for the patient. The time and effort required to maintain nutrition in a terminally ill or persistently comatose patient may well compromise the care of other patients.

Finally, the intent to withdraw artificial feeding must be to benefit the patient—by discontinuance of futile, burdensome measures that interfere with the process of dying.[14] It cannot simply be to hasten the death of the patient. This is a point on which the statements of two recent authoritative bodies agree. One is a statement issued by the AMA Council on Ethical and Judicial Affairs[15] and the other, a group assembled under the aegis of the Pontifical Academy of Sciences.

Both groups also agreed that under certain specific conditions, such as a persistent vegetative state in a brain-damaged patient, medical treatments that would be futile or burdensome could be discontinued. They disagreed, however, on the matter of nutrition and hydration. The AMA council, following court decisions, classified them as medical treatments that could be withdrawn on the same criteria as any other medical treatment. The Vatican group classified nutrition and hydration as "care" that must never be discontinued. On this point the Vatican group is in disagreement with the *Barber and Nejdl* case, the *Conroy* case, and decisions in the *Bartling* and *Bouvia* cases, to be discussed.

Another issue raised in this case is the possibility of moral conflict between members of the health care team. The nurse in the *Barber and Nejdl* case judged that the physicians were not providing the ordinary care that was customary in the hospital's intensive care unit. It was her objection that precipitated the court's intervention.

In our view of the matter, the nurse is also a guardian of the patient's welfare. She, also, is bonded to the patient by the principle of beneficence-in-trust. She, too, is a responsible moral agent. Her moral agency cannot be overridden by the physician. Indeed, if she believes a serious harm is being done, she is morally bound to object and take what measures she thinks morally required of her. A parallel situation occurred in the *Baby Doe*[16] case in Indiana, in which the pediatrician disagreed with the parents and the obstetrician, and the *Baby Jane Doe*[17] case in New York, in which a third party disagreed with the decision of the parents and the attending physician.

From the moral point of view we have taken, we cannot resolve the conflict simply by granting absolute decision-making authority to parents and physicians, as many would wish. Rather, we would hope that some resolution must be sought through discussion among members of the health care team.[18] If this fails, recourse to hospital ethics committees and, finally, the courts, is necessary.

While we do not think the courts are the right place to settle most moral conflicts, we believe they should be used when serious moral conflicts with significant consequences to patients are otherwise unresolvable. As we have pointed out in chapter 13, the court cannot settle the moral issue, but it does permit a decision to be made and action taken. Those who feel the court's decision is immoral are bound to disobey, but also to suffer the legal consequences.

IN RE BARTLING

William Bartling[19] was a seventy-year-old man with chronic obstructive lung disease who was admitted to a California hospital for treatment of depression and chronic back pain. When a chest X ray showed a new pulmonary nodule, a needle aspiration was performed and showed carcinoma of the lung. After the procedure Bartling required mechanical ventilation. Even though frequent attempts were made, he could not be weaned off the respirator over the next few months. He, and his wife and family, asked that he be removed from the respirator, but the physicians and the hospital administration refused this request.

When the case reached the lower courts, a deposition by the patient was videotaped and shown over CBS's "60 Minutes." When asked whether he wished to be removed from the respirator and whether he understood that he would die, the patient wrote yes. However, he did answer "no" to the question of whether he wanted to die. The judge then ruled that he was equivocating, even though the brief interview would have established the patient's wishes in this case. Yet caregivers pointed out that he often changed his mind, and that his clinical depression might possibly be reversible. The court did not explicitly deal with either of these considerations. This is a good instance of how the legal system does not deal directly with the specific nuances of decision making that make clinical judgment so difficult. The legal system in this case appeared to be naive and imprecise with respect to medical facts and values.

During the course of this case, Bartling appears to have been treated against his current preference, confirmed by his wife and family as consistent with his values. This problem was caused by hospital administrators, since the physicians eventually agreed to accept even the smallest legal uncertainty over withdrawing life-supporting treatment. Had their objection been made on moral grounds, it could have been admissible, as was the objection of the nurse. However, fear of suit is not a morally valid warrant for overriding the patient's wishes.

On the principle of beneficence-in-trust, the patient's preferences should have been checked more thoroughly with his perduring values. In particular, treatment for depression could have been instituted to eliminate or ameliorate a potentially reversible impediment to decision making. If, as it appears in retrospect, Bartling's wishes were perduring despite his depression, they should have been honored. On this point our discussion in chapter 13 about the dialogical model of the fiduciary doctor-patient relationship is relevant. Kapp and Lo comment on this decision in the same vein.[20]

IN RE CONROY

We have discussed the case of Claire C. Conroy[21] at several points throughout this book. She was senile, suffering from heart problems and chronic diabetes, and locked in a permanent fetal position. When the nursing home could no longer feed her orally, they inserted a nasogastric feeding tube. Her nephew objected, arguing on the basis of what we have called "presumed wishes" that his aunt would not have wanted this intervention. As the court deliberated, Conroy passed away with the tube in place. Nonetheless, the New Jersey Supreme Court decided to hear the case and made several important decisions.

First, in order to protect patients such as Conroy, who often do not have families present to make decisions, the court mandated that withdrawing life-supporting systems required consultation with two physicians and a state ombudsman official. The latter was charged with investigating each case of treatment withdrawal in elderly incompetent patients as cases of possible elder abuse. Stollerman[22] and Nevins[23] are among the physicians who objected. Both argued that physicians must be able to act in the best interest of the patient without such bureaucratic encumbrances.

On the whole, ethicists reacted favorably to the ruling. Since it is based on several principles we have defended, it is worth spelling these out. First, the court underlined the legal and ethical principle that, even when patients become incompetent, they do not lose their right to determine their care.

Second, through the three "tests" we have discussed elsewhere (chapter 4), the court established guidelines for proxy decision making: One can employ substituted judgment if based on evidence of such patient values (the subjective test). Next, one turns to the limited objective test by appeal to reliable evidence of wishes (what we have called presumed wishes—the fourth step of our hierarchy in chapter 13) and the calculation of burdens and benefits. Finally, one turns to the pure objective test (actually a form of medical indications and benefits-to-burdens calculus, with the added judgment that continued treatment would be cruel or cause undue pain).

The hierarchy we have proposed alters this last step a bit by indicating only that the physician may construct probable values that could lead to a decision to withdraw treatment without the necessity of demonstrating cruelty to continue such treatment (unless one were to count the "burdens" as being cruel).

The third principle in the *Conroy* case is also very important. It is the definitive legal statement that fluids and nutrition are to be considered medical treatments because they are food and water delivered medically. This means that they are as optional as other treatments considered to be "extraordinary" in the past. We have presented our view on this point in our discussion of the *Barber and Nejdl* case above.

To some, it appears that *Conroy* left open the possibility of moving the aged and senile into the category of dying patients, and then applying to them the ethical guidelines regarding withdrawing treatment from dying patients. We believe the *Conroy* case actually protects against that eventuality through its requirement of external evaluation of the case. In fact, the case resolution is built on presumed patient wishes. In this respect the principle of beneficence-in-trust would have led to the same conclusion.

IN RE BROPHY

Court cases continue to indicate the divergence of opinion about specific treatment decisions, especially about food and water.[24] This divergence is not different than that which might appear in clinical decision making, although convergence of social values and public opinion seems to occur more readily through highly dramatic court cases.

In the *Brophy*[25] case the court refused permission to remove a gastrostomy tube on the grounds that the patient was not terminal, the tube not a form of burdensome treatment, and the intent to hasten death was inadmissible. The opinion of the court turned on a distinction between withholding and withdrawing feedings that many find morally dubious. Also, seven ethicists testified. The judge was forced to pick from among their testimonies to support his conclusion, raising some new questions: What influence should an ethicist's testimony have on a legal decision? Should it have the same influence as that of an expert witness in medicine? Ethicists have testified in almost every court case in the past as well, and the literature of ethics finds its way into the opinions of judges. Further, is the judge qualified to decide among ethical opinions if such should conflict? If so, how much more qualified is the judge in this regard than the managing physician?

We would respond to the questions in this way: The ethicist must testify in court like any other expert—within the confines of his or her discipline. The discipline of ethics deals only with generally true statements. The certitude of ethics is a certitude Saint Thomas Aquinas called *ut in pluribus,* translated as "generally, for the most part." Hence, ethicists disagree on some points while agreeing on others. The influence an ethicist's opinions should have on legal decisions is therefore problematic. Ethics and law are different domains. The task of the court is to apply existing law in a particular case. The decision depends upon the facts in the case (in this circumstance the clinical data) and their relevance to a particular law or statute. Whether a particular action is morally defensible is a different question, and one that should not influence the interpretation of the law unless the infringement of morality under question is also an infringement of the law.

An ethicist's testimony in a court of law is therefore problematic unless the court's function is actually to decide what is morally right and good, rather than what is legally acceptable. As anyone versed in ethics might predict, the seven ethicists sometimes disagreed. The judge chose the ethical opinion he felt was correct. What criteria did he use to differentiate among the ethicists' opinions? If they were legal criteria, there was no need for the ethicists' testimony. If they were his own values, they would have no more validity than those of the ethicists. Presumably, the judge reached for "common moral principles" found in our culture. These are difficult to find, however. The problem we raise here bears more scrutiny.

We would have the same reservations about references to the recent opinion of the AMA Council on Ethical and Judicial Affairs in the *Bouvia* case and the *Jobes* case, presented below. With all due respect to the AMA's position and influence, its pronouncements do not have the force of law.

IN RE JOBES

In the *Jobes*[26] case the court ordered removal of a feeding ileostomy. Three neurologists diagnosed a permanent vegetative state; two others did not. The judge made his own examination, decided that the patient was, indeed, in a vegetative state, and alleged that the dissenting neurologists were influenced by their prior moral convictions. The moral status of the judge's clinical diagnosis (just as the *Brophy* judge's moral diagnosis discussed above) will certainly occasion controversy, as will his allegation that those who disagreed "tended to see signs of intelligence where no intelligence exists."[27]

This is a difficult case to reconcile with the principle of beneficence-in-trust. The patient's prognosis was essential in deciding what actions to take. Under the circumstance, a prognosis committee, as recommended by the *Quinlan* court, or a hospital ethics committee should be consulted. We do not believe that a judge is qualified to make the clinical diagnosis of a persistent vegetative state when even qualified neurologists disagree. In an analogous case, the *Torres* case, the Minnesota court recommended that the decision be checked with another ethics committee (as was done in the case) since some concern existed about negligence on the part of the first institution.[28] Consulting an ethics committee in such cases would be a sound practice.

IN RE BOUVIA

In the case of Elizabeth Bouvia,[29,30] many different court decisions on food and water fall into place. Bouvia was a twenty-six-year-old woman, almost quadriplegic from cerebral palsy, who entered a California hospital in 1983, saying that she wanted to starve to death. She also suffered from intense pain from arthritis, and did not feel that her life was worth living anymore. Unfortunately, she was unable to do much of anything about her condition or her own life, and was almost totally dependent on others for every bodily function. Her physicians and the county hospital believed that to honor her request for what is now called "assisted suicide" would have violated their duty to preserve life, involved them in a suicide attempt, which is not only illegal but immoral, and violated the rights of other patients who suffered from chronic illnesses. At that time a lower court rejected Bouvia's petition to prevent feeding against her will. The court also later authorized involuntary tube feedings.

Publicity entered this case in dramatic fashion. Disabled persons held vigils at the hospital to convince Bouvia to change her mind. Nurses took notes on her visitors and her telephone calls, all of which were later used against her in court. A national columnist offered to raise funds for her treatment. In the end, the superior court judge was asked to remove the feeding tube, with Bouvia promising through her lawyers to take food. The judge noted that "we all know Elizabeth pretty well right now." He held that she would not take food voluntarily, given her past history, and that the tube should stay in place. Throughout, an escalating cycle of confrontation, bitterness, and hostility developed. The partnership between doctor and patient we have articulated as necessary in making health care decisions completely breaks down in an adversarial relationship such as this, as Kapp and Lo have also observed.[31]

Bouvia's lawyers appealed the lower court decision and, in April of 1986, the Supreme Court of California issued its opinion. The court granted removal of a nasogastric feeding tube from Bouvia on the grounds that she was fully competent and had refused treatment. The court strongly asserted the doctrine of the right of privacy. It held that the right to determine treatment is not limited to comatose or terminally ill patients, that it is a personal rather than a legal or medical decision, and that whether or not it hastens death is immaterial. For the court, "It is incongruous, if not monstrous, for medical practitioners to assert the right to preserve life."[32] In making this decision the court disagreed with the earlier court, which argued that the state's interest and the physician's obligation to preserve life overrode Bouvia's right of privacy.

This 1986 decision is one of the bluntest defenses of patient autonomy as an absolute right, and the supposed constitutional right of privacy, equaled only by the libertarian arguments found in Engelhardt's book, *The Foundations of Bioethics,* which we discussed in chapter 2.[33] Both statements force physicians and ethicists to examine carefully what is gained and lost when autonomy is stressed to this extent. What is gained is an enhanced sense of freedom patients can enjoy, freedom at the very least from some of the pressures and confrontations Bouvia underwent. Second, personal control over proposed medical technology is accomplished. Also gained is a greater social respect for persons and their rights, especially those who are at the very edges of society because of their dependency on others or the nature of their illness (for example, AIDS victims).[34] Third, also gained is a social acceptance of commitments we suggest be part of the physician's moral duty to respect the right of patients to fashion their own values and execute decisions based on those values.

What is lost, however, when autonomy and privacy take absolute precedence over beneficence? First, the respect and mutuality of the doctor-patient relationship may suffer irreparable harm. In many of the cases examined so far, the bitterness and hostility arising from the moral conflicts destroy the therapeutic aim of the relationship. Second, as is so blatantly evident in the *Bouvia* decision, the conscience, motivation, and commitments of physicians to the good of their patients, and even perhaps their moral right to withdraw from a case when conscience requires, are questioned and even demeaned. The concurring opinion of Judge Compton in this case in effect reduces the health professional to a mere instrument of the patient's wishes. Such a view is surely deleterious to individual and social good. It ignores the bilaterality of the healing relationship and the moral agency of the physician. There is also the clear implication that the next logical move from the right of privacy is to the right to have active euthanasia "on demand." The moral, social, and political controversies of this decision are analogous to those of the *Roe vs. Wade* decision.

At stake in this important movement to respect the right of patients to refuse treatment is the limit placed on the physician's right to recommend, persuade, and advance the patient's good as he or she sees it. Traditionally, the physician's role included a teacher's role, upholding profoundly held values of the profession and society as well as the patient's own values.

In this case beneficence-in-trust requires attention to the values of Bouvia, who, indeed, has a legal right to refuse any treatments she wishes. Apparently, the reason she entered the hospital was to continue to receive pain medication and other forms of care while she carried out her plan to hasten her own death. This is a nontherapeutic aim with which a healing profession cannot cooperate. The value Bouvia sought is beyond the healing aims of medicine itself.

At issue, of course, was whether Elizabeth Bouvia was suffering from a terminal illness, not whether the quality of her life was worth sustaining. The patient knows best what quality of life can be tolerated and how it might be improved. Neither society nor the physician can make a quality-of-life determination for another person. What is really at issue here, then, is whether the patient can demand that a physician assist her in her direct intention to hasten death because, for her, life is intolerable. This is the problem of "assisted suicide."

The matter goes beyond the absolutization of the legal right of privacy and directly to the most fundamental beliefs about life and its meanings; just as in the *Roe vs. Wade* decision, this confrontation cannot be avoided. We would argue strenuously against the implications of Judge Compton's opinion that the health profession has an obligation to assist the patient to end her life. We would argue against the court opinion that the fact that the patient is not terminally ill is immaterial. We would hold that the physician cannot make decisions that directly have the intent of hastening or causing death.

Having said this, we reaffirm that moral right of a fully competent patient to refuse treatment. We believe Bouvia had a moral obligation to follow her own conscience, but so do her physician and the institution caring for her. We do not think it consistent with beneficence to assault a fully competent patient and treat her against her will. On the other hand, we do not think it permissible for a patient to require cooperation on the part of her medical attendants in an action they deem immoral.

Our argument is based on our belief that human life has a meaning beyond that which individuals or society may place on it. We do not hold life as an absolute in the sense that it must be sustained at all costs when it is futile to do so in a patient whose illness is terminal. We argue that interventions which merely prolong dying are not morally mandatory. But we do not agree that life can be discontinued at will when there is no terminal illness. We also argue that health and life are goods of the body, and that we have a responsibility to protect them in ourselves and others.

For us, the most difficult test of our principle of beneficence-in-trust is whether we would permit those who disagree with our assessment to cooperate with Bouvia in their intention to hasten her death. Having said we consider this immoral, are we prepared to insist that others who agree with Bouvia should be restrained from assisting her? In short, would we all possess free choice in such a case?

We would agree with Bouvia in withholding the tube in the first place. But once the tube was in place, we would not agree with its removal since the clear intent is to cause death by freeing her from her suffering. The distinction for us is between withdrawing treatment in a competent patient (which is active, direct, and formal cooperation in her death) and withholding treatment (which is passive, indirect, and material cooperation). Even if the tube were forcibly inserted in the first place, as it was in Bouvia's case, to remove it later would be to cooperate in a way that we do not think permissible.

We fully appreciate the objections that can be made to these distinctions. We propose to continue our examination of these dilemmas and urge our readers to do likewise. On purely philosophical grounds we might grant the inconsistency of our position. But we subscribe also to the theological source for morality, which in this instance we believe takes precedence. The relationship of a theocentric and anthropomorphic, philosophical, or theological ethics is a complex topic of greatest concern to us, but it is beyond the scope of this book.[35]

CORBETT VERSUS D'ALLESANDRO

A final case decision confirms the right of patients to decide about their treatment before they are dying, independent of a dying process, and when they face a terminal illness. In *Corbett v. D'Allesandro*[36,37] a Florida court ruled that artificial feeding and water could not be withdrawn from a patient because the state's living will statute expressly excluded artificial feeding and hydration. Yet in at least two states, courts have ruled that artificial fluids and nutrition, like any other life-prolonging technology, could be considered susceptible to withdrawal under the doctrine of substituted judgment or proportionality (California in *Barber and Nejdl* and *Bouvia,* and New Jersey in *Conroy*). Furthermore, statutes in some states cover food and water in the living will, while many others explicitly rule it out (Florida, Connecticut, Georgia, Illinois, Indiana, Iowa, Maine, Maryland, Missouri, New Hampshire, Oklahoma, Tennessee, Utah, Wisconsin, and Wyoming).

The decision in Florida was appealed. The final decision of the state supreme court was that it was unconstitutional for the state to exclude food and water delivered medically from the living will legislation. Consequently, patient values and wishes about this treatment are covered by the constitutional right of privacy. The food and water may be withdrawn.

As noted here, the processes of decision making for all patients, not just dying patients, should rest firmly on the grounds of patient values. But these should be subject to the process of negotiation and consensus should they butt against important values about the worth of human life and the dedication of the medical profession to preserving it. In the end, however, preserving life is not the final end of medicine. Rather, the end is healing. If healing is to involve the patient, as it must, then it must involve the patient's own values. Not all wishes of the patient are based on his or her values, however. So the development of a treatment plan requires constant negotiation and dialogue, not only about the medical realities, but also about the values to be protected in that plan. Physicians must be free to enter this negotiation with their own professional and personal values intact, and to withdraw from the process should the aim stretch beyond their own capacity to compromise.

CONCLUSION

Our effort to describe a middle road between paternalism and autonomy led to a description of beneficence-in-trust. In this chapter we described some significant court cases and how the principle of beneficence-in-trust lead to different determinations. Some general statements are possible as a result of this analysis.

1. The primary task of physicians is healing.
2. To that end, since one cannot heal by neglecting or overriding patient wishes, physicians must be stewards of patient values and preferences whenever possible.
3. When and if these values conflict with the medically indicated course of treatment, physicians' consciences must be protected such that, if negotiations about values threaten to destroy their life-affirming convictions, they are free, indeed duty bound, to withdraw from the case.
4. Conflicting court decisions simply portray the fact that the lines of negotiation about values, particularly the extent patient values can modify the healing aim of the relation, will vary from case to case, patient to patient, physician to physician, and culture to culture.
5. Thus, the stewardship of patient values is blocked on one hand by the prohibition against paternalism. On the other, it is blocked by the limits on patient autonomy a hierarchy of goods may impose on a case.
6. The search for common ethical principles to resolve dilemmas arising in conflicts is fruitless in a pluralistic society, as MacIntyre has argued to our satisfaction.[38]
7. The best resolution is not, as Engelhardt argues, enhancing individual freedoms to the point of destroying moral values in medicine,[39] but rather to articulate the life-affirming values of the medical profession not only as a basis for dialogue about values in the doctor-patient relation, but also as a protection for those health professionals who morally object to being forced to assist the suicide of their patients.
8. In this way, even though cultural pluralism cannot lead to an a priori assumption of values, some common values in the medical transaction can be formulated as a baseline for a new code of the healing professions.

We turn to this task in the last chapter.

16

A Medical Oath for the Post-Hippocratic Era

Over the last two decades, more change has taken place in medical ethics than ever before in its entire twenty-five-hundred-year history. The whole edifice of Hippocratic ethics has been shaken, and some parts of it dismantled. We are entering a post-Hippocratic era whose future is uncertain, one in which there is serious question about whether the medical profession can ever again be united under a common set of moral commitments.[1]

The task before the profession today is one of reconstruction—building a new ethics on elements from the past that are still viable, and discarding those elements that are not.[2] We believe that the principle of beneficence-in-trust that we have set forth in this book provides a foundation for commitments consistent with the best in the Hippocratic tradition and yet responsive to the needs of contemporary society.

Any attempt at reconstruction must take account of the forces of deconstruction that have been at work in Western society at least since the Enlightenment. Chief among them is the loss of moral consensus and the moral authority of religious institutions. The resulting moral diversity has been accentuated in our country in the last twenty years by the convergence of other forces—better public education, media exposure of the moral dilemmas in medical progress, the spread of consumerism and participatory democracy, a general mistrust of authority and experts, and, sadly, the undeniable moral defection of some physicians.[3]

As a result, patients and physicians cannot assume they will share any common set of moral values—especially about such fundamental matters as the source, meaning, and purpose of human life. They may find, instead, at a time when the most fateful decisions must be made, that they are moral adversaries. A legalistic rather than a fiduciary climate then comes to dominate many physician-patient relationships. Litigation and court decisions become the arena for the settlement of ethical disputes.

These same forces, of course, also divide the members of the healing professions. In medicine every one of the prescriptions and proscriptions of the Hippocratic oath has been questioned or openly violated: Abortion is no longer forbidden; confidentiality has been challenged as outmoded; direct euthanasia is proposed and even quietly practiced; and sexual relationships with patients are deemed therapeutic by some psychiatrists. Most of all, the benignly paternalistic image of the physician so characteristic of the Hippocratic ethos is everywhere under attack. Indeed, traditional medical ethics itself is perceived by some to be simply a mechanism for preserving professional power and privilege.[4,5]

As we have argued in this book, some of these changes are salubrious; others, of doubtful validity; and still others, morally untenable. We do not believe that universal agreement can be restored to medical ethics—if it ever really existed. But we do believe that many physicians are still deeply dedicated to the good of their patients, and that this is the bond that unites and inspires them as a profession despite differences they may have at more fundamental moral levels.[6,7]

We are also under no illusion that any single measure can undo the erosion of moral credibility from which the profession today suffers in many quarters. Nevertheless, we think an effort to reconstruct a code of ethics suitable to our times is in order for several reasons.

First, it is essential that the public know what commitments the profession will make to thier care, especially in areas where the Hippocratic oath and the code of the AMA are silent.[8] Then, such a code might reawaken the ideal of service in the ambivalent or passive members of the profession who need some reinforcement of their dedication to patient well-being. Lastly, there must be evidence that some physicians do not accept the dilution of patient advocacy in for-profit, entrepreneurial, and some prospective-payment plans.

It is our contention, following the line of argument this book has pursued, that the professional's moral credibility can be restored. To this end we offer a tentative declaration of commitment, not as a finished effort but as a stimulus to those who share our concern for the moral integrity of the profession and, more importantly, for the good of those it purports to serve.

We are by no means the first to make this attempt, nor will we be the last. Abrams has made an attempt that came to our attention after we began formulating our own.[9] Napodano has constructed a list of values important to the healing profession, which include dedication to serving the sick, truthfulness, beneficence, moral responsibility, respect for life from beginning to end, and other very important features. Although this list is not presented as an oath or declaration, Napodano's concern is to outline appropriate values, attitudes, and behavior for the modern physician.[10] Like the American Board of Internal Medicine's list of humanistic qualities of the internist, Napodano's primary interest is in teaching programs that emphasize the qualities physicians must possess.

Similarly, Bulger has prepared a new Hippocratic oath. Hippocrates (in his modern guise) reconstructs his old oath and develops it for the modern physician. Once again, truthfulness, commitment to needs, and recognition of the patient's values are predominant features.[11] The commitments we list are, therefore, not at all unique. They do, however, follow directly from the theory of beneficence-in-trust we have developed throughout this book.

Our declaration of commitment rests on three axioms: first, that the essence of a true profession lies in its public promise to act in certain ways required by the nature of its role in society; second, that the primary commitment of a true profession, distinguishing it from other human activities, is the higher degree of altruism it calls forth in the interest of those it serves; and, third, that the obligations of health professionals are grounded in the nature of illness, in faithfulness to their promise to help, and in the power to help that resides in professional knowledge and skill. The justification of these axioms has been the central task of the preceding chapters of this book.

A PHYSICIAN'S COMMITMENT TO PROMOTING THE PATIENT'S GOOD

I promise to fulfill the obligations I voluntarily assume by my profession to heal, and to help those who are ill. My obligations rest in the special vulnerability of the sick and the trust they must ultimately place in me and my professional competence. I therefore bind myself to the good of my patient in its many dimensions as the first principle of my professional ethics. In recognition of this bond, I accept the following obligations from which only the patient or the patient's valid surrogates can release me:

1. To place the good of the patient at the center of my professional practice and, when the gravity of the situation demands, above my own self-interest
2. To possess and maintain the competence in knowledge and skill I profess to have.
3. To recognize the limitations of my competence and to call upon my colleagues in all the health professions whenever my patient's needs require.
4. To respect the values and beliefs of my colleagues in the other health professions and to recognize their moral accountability as individuals.
5. To care for all who need my help with equal concern and dedication, independent of their ability to pay.
6. To act primarily in behalf of my patient's best interests, and not primarily to advance social, political, or fiscal policy, or my own interests.
7. To respect my patient's moral right to participate in the decisions that affect him or her, by explaining clearly, fairly, and in language under-

stood by the patient the nature of his or her illness, together with the
benefits and dangers of the treatments I propose to use.

8. To assist my patients to make choices that coincide with their own values or beliefs, without coercion, deception, or duplicity.

9. To hold in confidence what I hear, learn, and see as a necessary part of
my care of the patient, except when there is a clear, serious, and immediate danger of harm to others.

10. Always to help, even if I cannot cure, and when death is inevitable, to
assist my patient to die according to his or her own life plans.

11. Never to participate in direct, active, conscious killing of a patient,
even for reasons of mercy, or at the request of the state, or for any other
reason.

12. To fulfill my obligation to society to participate in public policy decisions affecting the nation's health by providing leadership, as well as
expert and objective testimony.

13. To practice what I preach, teach, and believe and, thus, to embody the
foregoing principles in my professional life.

CONCLUSION

There are obvious difficulties to the general acceptance of such an oath of commitment. It would be presumptuous at this time to expect such a statement to
replace extant oaths and codes. The obstacles are formidable given the lack of
consensus on moral principles in the profession and our society, particularly on
the primary ordering principle of medical ethics.

The major points or debate will undoubtedly focus on direct killing (euthanasia), abortion, and the degree of autonomy that should be permitted the patient.
We have left abortion out of this statement because we are seeking a declaration
that would be widely accepted. Notwithstanding these objections, there are portions of this oath that should appeal to all physicians, which follow logically on
the reinstatement of beneficence as the ordering principle for professional ethics.
We invite our readers to consider this amplification of our professional commitment as a means of meriting the trust patients must place in us and as a
recognition of the centrality of the patient in all clinical decisions.

Notes

PREFACE

1. E. D. Pellegrino and D. C. Thomasma, *A Philosophical Basis of Medical Practice* (New York: Oxford University Press, 1981).

CHAPTER 1

1. E. Cassell, "The Function of Medicine," *Hastings Center Report,* Vol. 7, No. 7 (1977), 16–19.
2. A. MacIntyre, *After Virtue* (Notre Dame: University of Notre Dame Press, 1983).
3. J. Dewey, *Theory of the Moral Life* (New York: Holt, Rinehart, & Winston, 1960).
4. G. Chaines, "Impatient with Medical Arrogance," *Chicago Tribune,* Point of View, Sec. 1 (May 6, 1983), p. 24.
5. President's Commission for the Study of Ethical Problems in Medicine and Biomedical and Behavioral Research, *Making Health Care Decisions: Volume I* (Washington, DC: U.S. Government Printing Office, 1983).
6. "Oath of Hippocrates," in *Hippocrates,* W. H. S. Jones, tr. Loeb Classical Library (Cambridge: Harvard University Press, 1972), Vol. 1, p. 289.
7. R. Branson, et al. "The Quinlan Decision," *Hastings Center Report,* Vol. 6, No. 1 (1976), 8–19.
8. Indiana General Assembly, House Enrolled Act No. 1830, Section F, 1984.
9. D. C. Thomasma, "The Basis of Medicine and Religion: Respect for Persons," *Linacre Quarterly,* Vol. 47, No. 2 (1980), 142–150.
10. Pellegrino and Thomasma, *A Philosophical Basis,* pp. 208, 214.
11. H. T. Engelhardt, Jr., *The Foundations of Bioethics* (New York: Oxford University Press, 1986).

12. J. Bergsma with D. C. Thomasma, *Health Care: Its Psychosocial Dimensions* (Pittsburgh: Duquesne University Press, 1982).

13. T. Beauchamp and L. McCullough, *Medical Ethics: The Moral Responsibility of Physicians* (Englewood Cliffs, NJ: Prentice-Hall, 1983). p. 84.

14. D. W. Brock, "Paternalism and Promoting the Good," in R. Sartorius, ed., *Paternalism* (Minneapolis: University of Minnesota Press, 1983), pp. 237–260.

15. L. H. Newton, "The Patient as Responsible Adult: Derivations and Consequences of the Revised Perspective," in D. O. Dahlstrom, D. T. Ozar, and L. Sweeney, eds., *Proceedings of the Fifty-Fifth Annual Meeting of the American Catholic Philosophical Association* Vol. LV (Washington, DC: American Catholic Philosophical Association, 1981), pp. 240–249.

16. R. M. Veatch, "Professional Medical Ethics: The Grounding of Its Principles," *Journal of Medicine and Philosophy,* Vol. 4, No. 1 (1979), 1–19. This position has been amplified in the last chapter of Veatch's later book, *A Theory of Medical Ethics* (New York: Basic Books, 1981).

17. P. Ramsey, *The Patient as Person* (New Haven: Yale University Press, 1970), pp. 5–32.

18. Veatch, *A Theory of Medical Ethics,* pp. 324–330.

19. Pellegrino and Thomasma, *A Philosophical Basis,* pp. 58–81; 77–78; 170–220.

20. R. Gillon, "More on Professional Ethics," editorial, *Journal of Medical Ethics,* Vol. 12, No. 2 (1986), 59–60.

21. E. D. Pellegrino, *Humanism and the Physician* (Knoxville, Tenn: University of Tennessee Press, 1979), p. 127.

22. J. Childress, *Priorities in Biomedical Ethics* (Philadelphia: Westminster Press, 1981), p. 14.

23. J. F. Childress, "Paternalism and Health Care," in W. L. Robinson and M. S. Pritchard, eds., *Medical Responsibility* (Clifton, NJ: Humana Press, 1979), pp. 15–27.

24. Metro-Goldwyn-Mayer presents Richard Dreyfus and John Cassavetes in *Whose Life Is It Anyway?,* a John Badham film. © 1981, Metro-Goldwyn-Mayer Film Co.

25. T. F. Ackerman, "Fooling Ourselves with Child Autonomy and Assent in Nontherapeutic Clinical Research," *Clinical Research,* Vol. 27, No. 5 (1979), 345–348.

26. G. Dworkin, "Paternalism," *The Monist,* Vol. 56, No. 1 (1972), 78.

27. J. S. Mill, *Utilitarianism; On Liberty; Essay on Bentham; Together with selected writings of Jeremy Bentham and John Austin,* M. Warnock, ed. (Cleveland: World, 1962), pp. 256–278.

28. G. Dworkin, "Autonomy and Behavior Control," *Hastings Center Report,* Vol. 6, No. 1 (1976), 23–28.

29. Cassell, "The Function of Medicine," 16–19.

30. C. M. Culver and B. Gert, *Philosophy in Medicine: Conceptual and Ethical Issues in Medicine and Psychiatry* (New York: Oxford University Press, 1982), pp. 126–135.

31. A. Buchanan, "Medical Paternalism," *Philosophy and Public Affairs,* Vol. 7 (1978), 370–390.

32. G. Dworkin, "Paternalism," in R. A. Wasserstrom, ed., *Morality and the Law* (Belmont, Calif: Wadsworth, 1971), p. 108.

33. J. Childress, *Who Should Decide? Paternalism in Health Care* (New York: Oxford University Press, 1982), p. 13.

34. Ibid., pp. 12–13

35. Ibid., p. 239.

36. Ibid., p. 32.

37. Ibid., p. 41.

38. Pellegrino and Thomasma, *A Philosophical Basis,* pp. 155–168.
39. L. St. Aubin, *Healing* (London: William Heinemann, 1983).
40. M. J. DeVries, "Healing and the Process of Healing," *Humane Medicine,* Vol. 1 (1985), 53–61. DeVries adds a fifth stage, restitution, to these four, arguing that the new tissue or new psychosocial makeup is reintegrated into the system as a whole.
41. E. D. Pellegrino, "Health Care: A Vocation to Justice and Love," in F. A. Eigo, ed., *The Professions in Ethical Context* (Villanova University: Proceedings of the Theology Institute of Villanova University, 1986), pp. 97–126.

CHAPTER 2

1. Newton, "The Patient as Responsible Adult," pp. 240–249.
2. Neither in the oath, nor the other deontological books, nor the whole body of the Hippocratic corpus is there evidence of an obligation to obtain patient consent or participation. Indeed, most of the direct references were to the contrary; see E. D. Pellegrino, "Toward a Reconstruction of Medical Morality: The Primacy of the Act of Profession and the Fact of Illness," *The Journal of Medicine and Philosophy,* Vol. 4, No. 1 (March 1979), 32–56.
3. J. Katz, *The Silent World of Doctor and Patient* (New York: Free Press, 1984).
4. E. D. Pellegrino, "Foreword: Thomas Percival, The Ethics Beneath the Etiquette," in T. Percival, *Medical Ethics, or a Code of Institutions and Precepts Adapted to the Professional Conduct of Physicians and Surgeons* (Birmingham: Classics of Medicine Library, 1985).
5. W. Hooker, *Physician and Patient* (New York: Backer and Scribner, 1849).
6. P. Lain-Entralgo, *La Medicina Hipocratica* (Madrid: Revista de Occidente, 1970).
7. P. Lain-Entralgo, *Doctor and Patient* (New York: World University Library, 1969).
8. E. Freidson, *Doctoring Together: A Study of Professional Social Control* (New York: Elsevier, 1975).
9. J. S. Mill, *On Liberty,* E. Rapaport, ed. (Indianapolis: Hackett, 1978), p. 6.
10. I. Illich, *Medical Nemesis* (New York: Pantheon, 1976).
11. L. S. Freshneck, *Physician and Public Attitudes on Health Care Issues* (Chicago: American Medical Association, 1984).
12. J. L. Berlant, *Profession and Monopoly* (Berkeley: University of California Press, 1985).
13. D. Thomasma, "The Goals of Medicine and Society," in D. H. Brock, ed., *The Culture of Biomedicine: Studies of Science and Culture* (Newark: University of Delaware Press, 1985), pp. 34–54.
14. E. J. Cassell, *The Healer's Art* (New York: J. B. Lippincott, 1976).
15. P. Bradley, "A Response to the March 1979 Issue of *The Journal of Medicine and Philosophy,*" *Journal of Philosophy* Vol. 5, No. 3 (1980), 213. See also Pellegrino and Thomasma, *A Philosophical Basis.*
16. E. J. Cassell, "Disease as an 'It': Concepts of Disease Revealed by Presentation of Symptoms," *Social Science and Medicine,* Vol. 10, Nos. 3/4 (1976), 143–146.
17. E. D. Pellegrino, "Being Ill and Being Healed: Some Reflections on the Grounding of Medical Morality," *Bulletin of the New York Academy of Medicine,* Vol. 56, No. 1 (1981), 70–79.
18. E. D. Pellegrino, "Moral Choice, the Good of the Patient, and the Patient's Good," in J. Moskop and L. Kopelman, eds., *Ethics and Critical Care Medicine* (Dordrecht: D. Reidel, 1985), pp. 117–136.

19. Thomasma, "The Basis of Medicine and Religion," 142–150.
20. D. C. Thomasma, "Professional and Ethical Obligations Toward the Aged," *Linacre Quarterly,* Vol. 48, No. 1 (1981), 73–80.
21. D. C. Thomasma, "The Context as a Moral Rule in Medical Ethics," *Journal of Bioethics,* Vol. 5, No. 1 (1984), 63–79.
22. H. T. Engelhardt, Jr., "Understanding Safe Traditions in the Context of Health Care: Philosophy as a Guide for the Perplexed," in M. E. Marty and K. L. Vaux, eds., *Health/Medicine and the Faith Traditions* (Philadelphia: Fortress Press, 1982), 163–184.
23. A. Soffer, "Searching Questions and Inappropriate Answers," commentary, *Archives of Internal Medicine,* Vol. 142, No. 6 (1982) 1117–1118.
24. T. Beauchamp and J. Childress, *Principles of Biomedical Ethics* (New York: Oxford University Press, 1979), pp. 56–57.
25. E. D. Pellegrino, "Treating the Patient as Person: Philosophical Groundings—Commentary on Alasdair MacIntyre," in E. J. Cassell and M. Siegler, eds., *Changing Values in Medicine* (Frederick, Md: University Publications of America, 1985), pp. 97–104.
26. D. C. Thomasma, "The Basis of Medicine and Religion," 142–150.
27. E. D. Pellegrino, Commencement Address, University of Illinois at the Medical Center, Chicago, June 6, 1980.
28. T. McGovern, "The Patient Comes First," *Forum of Medicine,* Vol. 3 (1980), 596–598.
29. E. D. Pellegrino, "The Healing Relationship: Architectonics of Clinical Medicine," in E. Shelp, ed., *The Clinical Encounter, The Moral Fabric of the Patient-Physician Relationship* (Dordrecht: D. Reidel, 1983), pp. 153–172.
30. F. J. Ingelfinger, "Arrogance," *New England Journal of Medicine,* Vol. 303, No. 26 (1980), 1507–1511.
31. Engelhardt, *Foundations of Bioethics.*
32. *Bartling v. Superior Court,* 209 Cal. Reptr. 70 (1984); *Bartling v. Glendale Adventist Medical Center,* 229 Cal. Rptr. 360 (1986).
33. *Elizabeth Bouvia v. Superior Court (Glenchur),* 225 Cal. Rptr. 297 (1986).
34. B. Lo, "The Bartling Case: Protecting Patients from Harm While Respecting Their Wishes," *Journal of the American Geriatrics Society,* Vol. 34, No. 1 (1986), 44–48.
35. E. D. Pellegrino, "Informal Judgments of Competence and Incompetence," in H. T. Engelhardt, Jr., M. A. Gardell, and E. E. Shelp, eds., *When Are Competent Patients Incompetent?* (Dordrecht: D. Reidel, in press).
36. E. H. Morreim, "Different Notions of Autonomy and Competence: Their Implications for Medicine and Public Policy," in H. T. Engelhardt, Jr., M. A. Gardell, and E. E. Shelp, eds., *When Are Competent Patients Incompetent?* (Dordrecht: D. Reidel, in press).
37. D. Thomasma, "The Context as a Moral Rule," 63–79.
38. L. Kopelman, "Teaching Commentary: The Case-Method and the Case-Method Fallacy," *Society for Health and Human Values Notes,* Vol. 15 (February 1985), 2–3.
39. L. McCullough and S. Wear, "Respect for Autonomy and Medical Paternalism Reconsidered," *Theoretical Medicine,* Vol. 6, No. 3 (1985), 295–308.
40. J. Childress, "Ensuring Care, Respect, and Fairness for the Elderly," *Hastings Center Report,* Vol. 14, No. 5 (1984), 31.
41. President's Commission for the Study of Ethical Problems in Medicine and Biomedical and Behavioral Research (Washington, DC: U.S. Government Printing Office) (multivolume Series).
42. Department of Health and Human Services, "Child Abuse and Neglect: Prevention

and Treatment Program: The Final Rule," *Federal Register,* Vol. 50, No. 72 (April 15, 1985), 14878–14901.

43. Engelhardt, *The Foundations of Bioethics.*
44. J. C. Murray, *We Hold These Truths* (New York: Sheed & Ward, 1960).
45. M. Angell, "The Baby Doe Rules," *New England Journal of Medicine,* Vol. 314, No. 10 (1986), 642–644. See also "Child Abuse and Neglect Prevention and Treatment Program: The Final Rule," *Federal Register,* Vol. 50, No. 72 (April 15, 1985), 14878–14901.
46. Cassell, *The Healer's Art.*
47. Childress, *Who Should Decide?*
48. Pellegrino, "Moral Choice," pp. 117–136.
49. W. K. Frankena, *Ethics* (Englewood Cliffs, NJ: Prentice-Hall, 1963).
50. G. Outka, *Agape: An Ethical Analysis* (New Haven: Yale University Press, 1972).
51. D. Ozar, "Social Ethics, the Philosophy of Medicine, and Professional Responsibility," *Theoretical Medicine,* Vol. 6, No. 3 (1985), 281–294.
52. M. Siegler, "Should Age Be a Criterion in Health Care?" *Hastings Center Report,* Vol. 5, No. 5 (1984), 24–27.
53. D. Thomasma, "Freedom, Dependency, and the Care of the Very Old," *Journal of the American Geriatrics Society,* Vol. 32, No. 12 (1984), 906–914.
54. J. N. Kvale, "Letter to the Editor," *Journal of the American Geriatrics Society,* Vol. 33, No. 6 (1985), 451–452.
55. R. A. McCormick, "Caring or Starving? The Case of Claire Conroy," *America* (April 6, 1985), 269–273.
56. T. Parsons, *The Social System* (New York: Free Press, 1964); T. Parsons, "The Sick Role and the Role of the Physician Reconsidered," *Milbank Memorial Fund Quarterly,* Vol. 53 (1975), 257–278.
57. S. Kelman, "Toward the Political Economy of Medical Care," *Inquiry,* Vol. 8 (1971), 30–38.
58. A. David, "Social and Role Constraints on Ethical Dilemmas in Hospitals," in D. Robbins and A. Dyer, eds., *Ethical Dimensions of Clinical Medicine* (Springfield, Ill: Charles C. Thomas, 1981), pp. 60–69.
59. Lain-Entralgo, *Doctor and Patient.*
60. Pellegrino and Thomasma, *A Philosophical Basis,* pp. 170–191.
61. Veatch, *A Theory of Medical Ethics,* p. 330.
62. D. Thomasma and A. Griffin, "Critical Care of Children: The Ethics of Using Contested and Expensive Medical Resources," *Linacre Quarterly,* Vol. 50, No. 4 (1983), 64–74.
63. G. Lundberg, "How Should Physicians Be Paid?" *Journal of the American Medical Association,* Vol. 254, No. 18 (1985), pp. 2638–2639.
64. M. Siegler, "Treating the Jobless for Free: Do Doctors Have a Special Duty?" *Hastings Center Report,* Vol. 13, No. 4 (1983), 12–14.
65. President's Commission for the Study of Ethical Problems in Medicine and Biomedical and Behavioral Research, *Securing Access to Health Care* (Washington, DC: U.S. Government Printing Office, 1983), p. 4.
66. D. C. Thomasma And E. D. Pellegrino, "Philosophy of Medicine as the Source for Medical Ethics," *Metamedicine,* Vol. 2, No. 1 (1981), 5–11.
67. M. Siegler, "Critical Illness: The Limits of Autonomy," *Hastings Center Report,* Vol. 7, No. 5 (1977), 12–15.
68. D. C. Thomasma, "Training in Medical Ethics: An Ethical Workup," *Forum on Medicine,* Vol. 1, No. 9 (1978), 33–36.
69. Katz, *The Silent World.*

70. T. Ackerman, "What Bioethics Should Be," *Journal of Medicine and Philosophy,* Vol. 5, No. 35 (1980), 260–275.

71. E. D. Pellegrino, "The Anatomy of Clinical Judgements: Some Notes on Right Reason and Right Actions," in H. T. Engelhardt, Jr., S. F. Spicker, and B. Towers, eds., *Clinical Judgement: A Critical Appraisal* (Dordrecht: D. Reidel, 1979), pp. 169–194.

72. E. D. Pellegrino, "The Virtuous Physician and the Ethics of Medicine," in E. Shelp, ed., *Virtue and Medicine: Explanations in the Character of Medicine* (Dordrecht: D. Reidel, 1985).

73. Aristotle *Nichomachean Ethics* bk. 1, ch. 8, 1099b, 1–2.

74. D. C. Thomasma, "Capstone Conference Workshops: Reflections on the State of the Art: Group 2," in *Teaching Ethics, The Humanities, and Human Values in Medical Schools: A Ten-Year Overview* (Washington, DC: Institute on Human Values in Medicine, 1982), pp. 66–79.

75. A. MacIntyre, "Why Is the Search for the Foundations of Ethics So Frustrating?" *Hastings Center Report,* Vol. 9, No. 4 (1979), 16–17.

76. F. J. Ingelfinger, "Arrogance," 1507–1511.

77. D. Callahan, "Shattuck Lecture—Contemporary Biomedical Ethics," *New England Journal of Medicine,* Vol. 302, No. 22 (1980), 1228–1233.

CHAPTER 3

1. P. Ramsey, *Ethics at the Edges of Life* (New Haven: Yale University Press, 1978).

2. Thomasma and Pellegrino, "Philosophy of Medicine," 5–11.

3. Pellegrino and Thomasma, *A Philosophical Basis,* pp. 119–152.

4. R. M. Veatch, *Death, Dying and the Biological Revolution* (New Haven: Yale University Press, 1976).

5. Ramsey, *The Patient as Person.*

6. Culver and Gert, *Philosophy in Medicine.*

7. Childress, *Who Should Decide?*

8. G. H. Stollerman, "Promoting Patient Autonomy: Looking Back," *Theoretical Medicine,* Vol. 5, No. 1 (1984), 9–16.

9. R. A. McCormick, "Experimentation in Children: Sharing in Sociality," *Hastings Center Report,* Vol. 6, No. 6 (1976), 41–46.

10. Ramsey, *Ethics at the Edges of Life.*

11. R. M. Veatch, "Interns and Residents on Strike," *Hastings Center Report,* Vol. 5, No. 6 (1975), 7–8.

12. Veatch, *A Theory of Medical Ethics,* pp. 214–226.

13. Thomasma and Griffin, "Critical Care of Children," 64–74.

14. Childress, *Priorities in Biomedical Ethics.*

15. E. D. Pellegrino and D. C. Thomasma, "Response to Our Commentators," *Metamedicine,* Vol. 2, No. 1 (1981), 43–51.

16. K. Nielsen, "On Being Skeptical About Applied Ethics," in T. Ackerman et al., eds., *Clinical Medical Ethics: Exploration and Assessment* (Lanham, Md: University Press of America, 1987), pp. 95–116.

17. MacIntyre, *After Virtue.*

18. R. S. Hartman, *The Structure of Value* (Carbondale, Ill: Southern Illinois University Press, 1967).

19. G. Marcel, "The Existential Fulcrum," in *The Mystery of Being* (Chicago: Henry Regnery, 1960), p. 123.

20. Engelhardt, *The Foundation of Bioethics.*

21. Ibid., p. 80.
22. Ibid., p. 84.
23. Ibid., p. 86.
24. H. T. Englehardt, Jr., "A Demand to Die," *Hastings Center Report*, Vol. 15, No. 3 (1975), 47.
25. See the excellent analysis of this and other points provided by E. H. Loewy's review, "Not by Reason Alone: A Review of Englehardt's *Foundations of Bioethics,*" *Journal of Medical Humanities and Bioethics,* Vol. 8 (1987), 67–72.
26. R. Veatch, "Autonomy's Temporary Triumph," *Hastings Center Report,* Vol. 14, No. 5 (1984), 41.
27. D. Callahan, "Autonomy: A Moral Good, Not a Moral Obsession," *Hastings Center Report,* Vol. 14, No. 5 (1984), 41.
28. R. Morison, "The Biological Limits on Autonomy," *Hastings Center Report,* Vol. 14, No. 5 (1984), 43–49.
29. D. Jackson and S. Youngner, "Patient Autonomy and 'Death with Dignity,'" *New England Journal of Medicine,* Vol. 301, No. 8 (1979), 404–408.
30. *In the matter of Claire C. Conroy,* 98 N.J. 321; 486 A. 2d 1209 (N.J. 1985).
31. P. Marzuk, "The Right Kind of Paternalism," *New England Journal of Medicine,* Vol. 313, No. 23 (1985), 1474–1476.

CHAPTER 4

1. H. Brody, "The Physician-Patient Relationship," *Theoretical Medicine,* in press.
2. R. Veatch, "The Hippocratic Ethic Is Dead," *The New Physician* (September 1984), 48.
3. C. Fried, *Right and Wrong* (Cambridge: Harvard University Press, 1979).
4. Veatch, "Professional Medical Ethics," 1–19.
5. Veatch, *A Theory of Medical Ethics.*
6. Veatch, "The Hippocratic Ethic Is Dead," 48.
7. Pellegrino, "Toward a Reconstruction of Medical Morality," 32–56.
8. Brody, "The Physician-Patient Relationship." Brody proposes a way to salvage the contract model by appeal to the "original position" in the writings of John Rawls. In this view the contract does not necessarily have to occur in the real world. Instead, it occurs in an ideal one. Although he thinks this notion needs much more rigorous work, Brody thinks enough of it to call it a "contractarian model"—a model in which the negotiators are rational and disinterested parties.
9. Katz, *The Silent World.*
10. H. Moody, "Paternalism and Autonomy in Long-Term Care: Are They in Conflict?" Project approved by the Retirement Research Foundation, Park Ridge, Illinois, for the period 12/85 to 6/86.
11. Ibid., p. 7.
12. F. Ingelfinger, "The Unethical in Medical Ethics," *Annals of Internal Medicine,* Vol. 83, No. 2 (1975), 264–269.
13. D. G. Smith and L. Newton, "Physician and Patient: Respect for Mutuality," *Theoretical Medicine,* Vol. 5, No. 1 (1984), 43–60. Smith and Newton observe that any attempt to reduce the doctor-patient relationship to a system of rules and regulations is one that tries to render that interaction "doctor-proof." In this rendering, physicians would participate in what is considered an ethically optimal relationship solely on the basis of moral principles and following the rules.
14. MacIntyre, *After Virtue.*

15. M. Siegler, "Searching for Moral Certainty in Medicine: A Proposal for a New Model of the Doctor-Patient Encounter," *Bulletin of the New York Academy of Medicine,* Vol. 57, No. 1 (1981), 56–69. Siegler acknowledges in a final note his debt to Stephen Toulmin in developing his model. In this regard see S. Toulmin, "The Tyranny of Principles," *Hastings Center Report,* Vol. 11, No. 6 (1981), 31–39.
16. Plato, as translated and cited by L. D. Weatherhead, *Psychology, Religion and Healing* (London: Hodder & Stoughton, 1951), p. 112. Also see K. A. Yonge, "The Philosophic Basis of Medical Practice. Part I: Body and Mind," *Humane Medicine,* Vol. 1 (March 1985), 25–29 and J. Bergsma, "Loyaal met de patient," *Metamedica,* Vol. 62 (1983), 202–211.
17. A. Jonsen and A. Jameton, "Social and Political Responsibilities of Physicians," *Journal of Medicine and Philosophy,* Vol. 2, No. 4 (1977), 376–400.
18. Pellegrino and Thomasma, *A Philosophical Basis.*
19. C. Fried, *Medical Experimentation: Personal Integrity and Social Policy* (New York: Elsevier, 1974), p. 77. Also see the development of this concept and its importance for the self-definition of the health professional in G. Graber, A. Beasley, and J. Eaddy, *Ethical Analysis of Clinical Medicine: A Guide to Self-Evaluation* (Baltimore: Urban & Schwarzenburg, 1985), pp. 118–123.
20. L. Kass, "Ethical Dilemmas in the Care of the Ill: What Is the Patient's Good?" *Journal of the American Medical Association,* Vol. 244, No. 17 (1980), 1946.
21. American Board of Internal Medicine, "Evaluation of Humanistic Qualities in the Internist," *Annals of Internal Medicine,* Vol. 99, No. 5 (1983), 720–724.
22. E. Pellegrino, and A. A. Pellegrino, "Scribonius Largus: The Stoic Origins of Medical Humanism," in *Literature and Medicine,* forthcoming.
23. *In the matter of Claire C. Conroy.*
24. S. Braithwaite and D. C. Thomasma, "New Guidelines on Foregoing Life-Sustaining Treatment in Incompetent Patients: An Anti-Cruelty Policy," *Annals of Internal Medicine,* Vol. 4, No. 5 (1986), 711–715.
25. Beauchamp and McCullough, *Medical Ethics,* pp. 50–51.
26. E. H. Morreim, "Cost Containment: Issues of Moral Conflict and Justice for Physicians," *Theoretical Medicine,* Vol. 6, No. 3 (1985), 257–279.
27. K. O'Rourke, *Medical Ethics: Common Ground for Understanding* (Saint Louis: Catholic Health Association, 1986), p. 16.
28. H. L. Smith and L. Churchill, *Professional Ethics and Primary Care Medicine* (Durham, NC: Duke University Press, 1986), p. 3.
29. S. Hauerwas, *Suffering Presence: Theological Reflections on Medicine, the Mentally Handicapped, and the Church* (Notre Dame: Notre Dame University Press, 1986), p. 6.

CHAPTER 5

1. Thomasma and Pellegrino, "Philosophy of Medicine," 5–11.
2. K. Sadegh-zadeh, "Normative Systems and Medical Metaethics. Part I: Value Kinematics, Health, and Disease," *Metamedicine,* Vol. 2, No. 1 (1981), 75–119.
3. Pellegrino and Thomasma, *A Philosophical Basis,* pp. 207–210.
4. E. D. Pellegrino, "Autonomy and Coercion in Disease Prevention and Health Promotion," *Theoretical Medicine,* Vol. 5, No. 4 (1984), 83–91.
5. L. Thomas, *Lives of a Cell* (New York: Viking, 1974).
6. Ozar, "Social Ethics," 281–294.

7. H. T. Engelhardt, Jr., "The Disease of Masturbation: Values and the Concept of Disease," in A. Caplan, ed., *Concepts of Health and Disease* (Reading, Mass: Addison-Wesley, 1981), pp. 31–45.
8. Smith and Churchill, *Professional Ethics.*
9. Ramsey, *The Patient as Person.*
10. Bergsma with Thomasma, *Health Care.*
11. A. Goldman, *The Moral Foundations of Professional Ethics* (Totowa, NJ: Rowman & Littlefield, 1980), pp. 156–229.
12. A. Goldman, "Authority, Autonomy, and Institutional Norms," *Perspective on the Professions* (Bulletin), Vol. 3 (March/June 1983), 1–5.
13. Ibid., p. 2.
14. K. Kipnis, "Unethical Professionalism: Alan Goldman's Foundations of Professional Ethics," *Perspective on the Professions* (Bulletin), Vol. 3 (March/June 1983), 10.
15. D. Luban, "Professional Ethics in a World Without Trumps," *Perspective on the Professions* (Bulletin), Vol. 3 (March/June 1983), 3.
16. R. Dworkin, *Taking Rights Seriously* (Cambridge: Harvard University Press, 1977).
17. Childress, *Who Should Decide?*
18. Veatch, "Professional Medical Ethics," 1–19.
19. Dworkin, *Taking Rights Seriously,* pp. 273–274.
20. Ibid., p. xi (our emphasis).
21. Ibid., p. 191.
22. Ibid., p. 204.
23. American Board of Internal Medicine, "Evaluation of Humanistic Qualities," 720–724.

CHAPTER 6

1. Brock, "Paternalism and Promoting the Good."
2. E. L. Erde, "The Place of the Good in the Science and Art of Medicine," *Man and Medicine,* Vol. 3, No. 2 (1978), 89–100.
3. Pellegrino and Thomasma, *A Philosophical Basis.*
4. Some of the relevant texts are Aristotle *Nicomachean Ethics,* bks. I and X.
5. Aristotle *Rhetoric,* bk. 1, ch. 5, 1361b5. See H. Veatch, "Telos and Teleology in Aristotelian Ethics, "In D. O'Meara, ed., *Studies in Aristotle* (Washington, DC: Catholic University of America Press, 1981), pp. 279–296.
6. K. V. Wilkes, "The Good Man and the Good for Man in Aristotle's Ethics," in A. O. Rorty, ed., *Essays on Aristotle's Ethics* (Berkeley: University of California Press, 1980), pp. 341–358.
7. N. P. White, "Goodness and Human Aims in Aristotle's Ethics," in D. O'Meara, ed., *Studies in Aristotle* (Washington, DC: Catholic University of America Press, 1981), pp. 225–246.
8. W. F. R. Hardie, "The Final Good in Aristotle's Ethics," in J. M. E. Moravcsik, ed., *Aristotle: A Collection of Critical Essays* (Garden City, NY: Anchor Books, 1967), pp. 296–322.
9. Ibid., p. 321.
10. R. B. Perry, *General Theory of Value* (New York: Longmans, Green, 1926).
11. White, "Goodness and Human Aims."
12. Aristotle, *Protrepticus,* in *Protrepticus, A Reconstruction,* A. H. Chroust, tr. (Notre Dame: University of Notre Dame Press, 1964), fr. 24, p. 11.
13. Pellegrino, "Autonomy and Coercion," 83–91.

14. Aristotle *Rhetoric* bk. 1, ch. 5, 1361b 3–4.
15. Aristotle *Nicomachean Ethics* bk. I, ch. 6, 1097a 6–13.
16. Erde, "The Place of the Good."
17. Pellegrino, "Toward a Reconstruction of Medical Morality," 32–56.
18. Ramsey, *Ethics at the Edges of Life,* pp. 189–227.
19. R. B. Brandt, *A Theory of the Good and the Right* (Oxford; Clarendon, 1979).
20. R. G. Olson, "The Good," in P. Edwards, ed., *The Encyclopedia of Philosophy* (New York: Macmillian and The Free Press, 1972), pp. 367–370.
21. Frankena, *Ethics,* pp. 63–77; 80–98.
22. Brock, "Paternalism and Promoting the Good."
23. *In the matter of Shirley Dinnerstein,* 380 N.E. 2d 134 (1978).
24. L. Lavelle, "The Problem of Evil," in J. J. Kockelmans, ed., *Contemporary European Ethics* (New York: Anchor Books, 1972), p. 18.
25. M. Abram, "To Curb Medical Suits," New York *Times* Monday, March 31, 1986, sec. 1, p. 19.
26. D. C. Thomasma, "Hospital Ethics Committees and Hospital Policy," *Quality Review Bulletin,* July 19, 1985, pp. 204–209.
27. A. Jonsen, M. Siegler, and W. Winslade, *Clinical Ethics: A Practical Approach to Ethical Decisions in Clinical Medicine* (New York: Macmillan, 1982), pp. 6–7.
28. Thomasma, "Hospital Ethics Committees."
29. Pellegrino and Thomasma, *A Philosophical Basis,* pp. 244–265.
30. Interview with De Vries as reported in R. Bazell, "Transplants on Trial," Forum/ Essay Cleveland *Plain Dealer* (February 7, 1985). p. 5b.
31. Interview with William Schroeder's wife as quoted in "Bionic Bill Fights for Life One Year Later," *U.S.A. Today* (November 14, 1985), pp. 1–2.
32. Childress, *Who Should Decide?* pp. 16–22.

CHAPTER 7

1. E. Shelp, ed., *Beneficence in Health Care* (Dordrecht: D. Reidel, 1982).
2. Lain-Entralgo, *La Medicina Hipocratica.*
3. Pellegrino and Thomasma, *A Philosophical Basis,* pp. 155–169.
4. *In the matter of Karen Quinlan,* 70 N.J. 10, 44; 355 A. 2d 647, cert. den., 429 U.S. 922; 50 L. Ed. 2d 289 (N.J. 1976).
5. *In the matter of Claire C. Conroy.*
6. M. Nevins, "Big Brother at the Bedside," *New Jersey Medicine,* Vol. 82 (1985), 950–952.
7. Braithwaite and Thomasma, "New Guidelines" 711–715.
8. R. Pearlman and A. Jonsen, "The Use of Quality-of-Life Consideration in Medical Deicison Making," *Journal of the American Geriatrics Society,* Vol. 33, No. 5 (1985), 348.
9. R. Pearlman and J. Speer, Jr., "Quality-of-Life Considerations in Geriatric Care," *Journal of the American Geriatrics Society,* Vol. 31, No. 2 (1983), 113–130.
10. D. Hilfiker, "Allowing the Debilitated to Die: Facing Our Ethical Choices," *New England Journal of Medicine,* Vol. 308, No. 12 (1983), 716–719.
11. A. Wagner, "Cardiopulmonary Resuscitation in the Aged: A Prospective Survey," *New England Journal of Medicine,* Vol. 310, No. 17 (1984), 1129–1130.
12. S. Bedell and T. Delbanco, "Choices About Cardiopulmonary Resuscitation in the Hospital: When Do Physicians Talk with Patients?" *New England Journal of Medicine,* Vol. 310, No. 17 (1984), 1089–1093.

13. R. Goldman, "Ethical Confrontations in the Incapacitated Aged," *Journal of the American Geriatrics Society,* Vol. 29, No. 6 (1981), 241–245.
14. President's Commission for the Study of Ethical Problems in Medicine and Biomedical and Behavioral Research: *Deciding to Forego Life-Sustaining Treatment: Ethical, Medical, and Legal Issues in Treatment Decisions* (Washington, DC: U.S. Government Printing Office, 1983).
15. D. Thomasma, "Philosophical Reflections on a Rational Treatment Plan," *Journal of Medicine and Philosophy,* Vol. 11, No. 2 (1986), 157–165.
16. Ramsey, *Ethics at the Edges of Life.*
17. S. Levey, "Richard McCormick and Proportionate Reason," *Journal of Religious Ethics,* Vol. 13, No. 2 (1985), 258–278.
18. R. Veatch, "What Is a 'Just' Health Care Policy?" in R. Veatch and R. Branson, eds., *Ethics and Health Policy* (Cambridge: Ballinger, 1976), pp. 127–153.
19. N. Daniels, "Am I My Parent's Keeper?" in President's Commission for the Study of Ethical Problems in Medicine and Biomedical and Behavioral Research, *Securing Access to Health Care* (Washington, DC: U.S. Government Printing Office, 1983), Appendix K, Vol. II, pp. 265–291.

CHAPTER 8

1. P. Lain-Entralgo, "What Does the Word 'Good' Mean in 'Good Patient'" in E. J. Cassell and M. Siegler, eds., *Changing Values in Medicine* (Frederick, Md.: University Publications of America, 1979), pp. 127–144.
2. T. Parsons, "Definitions of Health and Illness in Light of American Values and Social Structure," in A. Caplan, H. T. Engelhardt, and J. J. McCartney, eds., *Concepts of Health and Disease* (Reading, Mass: Addison-Wesley, 1981), pp. 57–86.
3. G. Glazer, "The 'Good' Patient," *Nursing and Health Care,* Vol. 11, No. 3 (1981), 144–164.
4. P. P. Bhanumathi, "Nurses' Conception of 'Sick Role' and 'Good Patient' Behaviour: A Cross-Cultural Comparison," *International Nursing Review,* Vol. 24, No. 1 (1977), 20–24.
5. I. Gladkij, "Soucasna predstava to veastnostich Dobreho pacienta a jeji teoreticky a practicky uyznam" [Contemporary Ideas on the Properties of a 'Good' Patient and Their Theoretical and Practical Importance], *Casopis Iekaru Ceskych,* Vol. 114 (1974), 702–706.
6. E. Freidson, *Patients' Views of Medical Practice* (New York: Russell Sage, 1961).
7. M. T. Westbrook, L. A. Nordholm, and J. E. McGee, "Cultural Differences in Reaction to Patient Behavior: A Comparison of Swedish and Australian Health Professionals," *Social Science and Medicine,* Vol 19, No. 9 (1984), 939–947.
8. J. D. Wasserman, "The Neglected Good Patient," *Dental Management,* Vol. 10, No. 11 (1970), 99–100.
9. A. P. Chesney et al. "Physician-Patient Agreement on Symptoms as a Predictor of Retention in Outpatient Care," *Hospital and Community Psychiatry,* Vol. 34, No. 8 (1983), 737–739.
10. B. Udell and R. K. Hornstra, "Three Utilization Styles at an Urban Mental Health Center," *Hospital and Community Psychiatry,* Vol. 28, No. 9 (1977), 700–702; B. Udell and R. K. Hornstra, "Good Patients and Bad. Therapeutic Assets and Liabilities," *Archives of General Psychiatry,* Vol. 32, No. 12 (1975), 1533–1537; and R. K. Hornstra and B. Udell, "Patterns of Psychiatric Utilization by Diagnosed Schizophrenics in the Kansas City Area," *Schizophrenia Bulletin,* Vol. 9 (1974), 133–147.

11. E. Freidson, *Profession of Medicine: A Study of The Sociology of Applied Knowledge* (New York: Dodd, Mead, 1970).

12. E. Goffman, *Asylums* (Garden City, NJ: Doubleday Anchor, 1961), pp. 341–342.

13. A. Cartwright, *Human Relations and Hospital Care* (London: Routledge & Kegan Paul, 1964).

14. J. Lorber, "Good Patients and Problem Patients: Conformity and Deviance in a General Hospital," *Journal of Health and Social Behavior,* Vol. 16, No. 2 (1975), 214.

15. J. Childress and M. Siegler, "Metaphors and Models of Doctor-Patient Relationships: Their Implications for Autonomy," *Theoretical Medicine,* Vol. 5, No. 1 (1984), 17–36.

16. L. Edelstein, "The Professional Ethics of the Greek Physician," in O. Temkin, ed., *Ancient Medicine: Selected Papers of Ludwig Edelstein* (Baltimore: Johns Hopkins University Press, 1967), pp. 319–348.

17. Veatch, *Death, Dying and the Biological Revolution.*

18. Freidson, *Doctoring Together.*

19. Bergsma with Thomasma, *Health Care.*

20. Veatch, *A Theory of Medical Ethics.*

21. Ramsey, *The Patient as Person.*

22. W. May, "Who Cares for the Elderly?" *Hastings Center Report,* Vol. 12, No. 6 (1982), 31–37.

23. Ramsey, *Ethics at the Edges of Life.*

24. C. Whitbeck, "On the Aims of Medicine: Comment on 'Philosophy of Medicine as the Source for Medical Ethics,'" *Metamedicine,* Vol. 2, No. 1 (1981), 35–41.

25. Pellegrino and Thomasma, *A Philosophical Basis,* pp. 119–152.

26. Siegler, "Treating the Jobless for Free" 12–14.

27. Katz, *The Silent World.*

28. American Medical Association, *Code of Ethics* (New York: Academy of Medicine, 1848), ch. 1, article II, no. 4.

29. Ibid.

30. D. Renshaw, "Patient's Secrets," *Physician and Patient,* Vol. 2, No. 9 (1983), 58–67.

31. M. Walfoort, "The Proper Guardian: Medical Care Decisions for Fatally Ill Children," *Forum,* Vol. 16, No. 2 (1982), 131–179; B. R. Grumet, "Just What the Doctor Ordered: The Role of Unconventional Therapy in the Treatment of Cancer in Minors," *Family Law Quarterly,* Vol. 14, No. 2 (1980), 63–98; E. Goodman, "What Doctors Say, What the Parents Want," Washington *Post,* January 27, 1979, p. A3.; and *Custody of a minor,* 379 N.E. 2d, 1053 (1978).

32. S. Gorovitz and A. MacIntyre, "Toward a Theory of Medical Fallibility," *Journal of Medicine and Philosophy,* Vol. 1, No. 1 (1976), 51–71.

33. Seneca *De Beneficiis* (Norwood, NJ: W. J. Johnson, 1974).

34. American Medical Association, *Code of Ethics; Adopted May 1847* (Philadelphia: Collins, 1848).

CHAPTER 9

1. G. Santayana, *Dominations and Powers, Reflections on Liberty, Society and Government* (New York: Scribner, 1951), p. 3.

2. MacIntyre, *After Virtue.*

3. M. Aurelius "Meditations," VI, 48, in W. J. Oates, ed., *The Stoic and Epicurean Philosophers* (New York: Modern Library, 1957).

4. P. Geach, *The Virtues* (Cambridge, England: Cambridge University Press, 1977).
5. J. D. Wallace, *Virtues and Vices* (Ithaca, NY: Cornell University Press, 1978).
6. W. K. C. Guthrie, *Socrates* (Cambridge, England: Cambridge University Press, 1971).
7. P. Foot, *Virtues and Vices* (Berkeley, Calif: University of California Press, 1978).
8. A. Kenny, *The Aristotelian Ethics* (Oxford: Clarendon, 1978).
9. J. Pieper, *The Four Cardinal Virtues* (Notre Dame: Notre Dame University Press, 1966).
10. R. Sokolowski, *The God of Faith and Reason* (Notre Dame: University of Notre Dame, 1982).
11. Shelp, ed., *Beneficence and Health Care.*
12. E. Shelp, ed., *Justice and Health Care* (Dordrecht: D. Reidel, 1981).
13. G. H. Von Wright, *The Varieties of Goodness* (New York: Humanities Press, 1965).
14. E. Shelp, ed., *Virtue and Medicine: Explorations in the Character of Medicine* (Dordrecht: D. Reidel, 1985).
15. MacIntyre, *After Virtue,* p. 245.
16. Pellegrino, "Toward a Reconstruction of Medical Morality," 32–56.
17. Pellegrino, "The Anatomy of Clinical Judgments," pp. 169–194.
18. F.M. Cornford, *Before and After Socrates* (Cambridge, England: Cambridge University Press, 1932).
19. A. E. Taylor, *Socrates: The Man and His Thought* (New York: Doubleday, 1953).
20. Guthrie, *Socrates.*
21. L. Versenyi, *Socratic Humanism* (New Haven: Yale University Press, 1963).
22. J. Gould, *The Development of Plato's Ethics* (New York: Russell & Russell, 1972).
23. Plato *Republic,* 351a.
24. Ibid., 444e.
25. Aristotle *Nicomachean Ethics,* bk. 1, ch. 8, 1099a, 10–11.
26. Ibid., bk. 1, ch. 8, 1099a, 10–11.
27. Ibid., bk. 2, ch. 1, 1103 a, 14–18.
28. Ibid., bk. 2, ch. 6, 1106a, 13–14.
29. Ibid., bk. 2, ch. 6, 1106a, 22–24.
30. W. D. Ross, *Aristotle: A Complete Exposition of His Works and Thought* (New York: Meridian, 1959), p. 215.
31. Aristotle *Nicomachean Ethics,* bk. 2, ch. 6, 1106a, 15–17.
32. Ibid., bk. 2, ch. 4, 1105a, 31–35.
33. Ibid., bk. 2, ch. 4, 1105a, 31–35.
34. Ibid., bk. 2, ch. 4, 1105b, 2–5.
35. MacIntyre, *After Virtue,* p. 166.
36. F. C. Copleston, *Aquinas* (Harmondsworth, Middlesex: Penguin, 1959), pp. 208–209.
37. Saint Thomas Aquinas, *Summa Theologica* I. IIi, Q57, a.4.
38. Saint Thomas Aquinas, *Commentary on the Virtues* 11, 5.
39. Ibid.
40. J. Maritain, *Art and Scholasticism with Other Essays* (New York: Scribner, 1947), p. 8.
41. Pieper, *The Four Cardinal Virtues.*
42. S. Hauerwas, *A Community of Character* (Notre Dame: University of Notre Dame Press, 1981).
43. C. S. Lewis, *Mere Christianity* (New York: Macmillan, 1952), pp. 76–77.
44. G. Engel, "The Clinical Application of Biopsychosocial Models," *American Journal of Psychiatry,* Vol. 137, No. 5 (1980), 535–544.
45. Von Wright, *The Varieties of Goodness,* pp. 139–140.
46. MacIntyre, *After Virtue,* p. 178.

47. Aristotle *Rhetoric,* in J. Barnes, ed., *The Complete Works of Aristotle* (Princeton: Princeton University Press, 1984).

48. Plato *Meno,* 79b–d, in B. Jowett, ed., *The Dialogues of Plato* (New York: Random House, 1937).

49. W. E. Frankena, "Beneficence in an Ethics of Virtue," in E. Shelp, ed., *Beneficence and Health Care* (Dordrecht: D. Reidel, 1982), p. 65.

50. Pellegrino and Pellegrino, "Scribonius Largus."

51. General Assembly of the World Medical Association, *Declaration of Geneva,* 1948.

52. American Board of Internal Medicine, "Evaluation of Humanistic Qualities," 720–724.

53. J. P. Reeder, Jr., "Beneficence, Supererogation, and Role Duty," in E. Shelp, ed., *Beneficence and Health Care* (Dordrecht: D. Reidel, 1982).

54. A. Jonsen, "Watching the Doctor," *New England Journal of Medicine,* Vol. 308, No. 25 (1983), 1531–1535.

55. Edelstein, "The Professional Ethics of the Greek Physician."

CHAPTER 10

1. H. Cushing, *Consecratio Medici and Other Papers* (Boston: Little, Brown, 1928), pp. 3–13.

2. Ibid., p. 4.

3. Ibid.

4. Edelstein, "The Professional Ethics of the Greek Physician," pp. 319–348.

5. C. C. Havihurst, "Competition in Health Services: Overview, Issues and Answers," *Vanderbilt Law Review,* Vol. 34, No. 117 (1981), 1117–1158.

6. Veatch, *A Theory of Medical Ethics.*

7. B. Weiser, "As They Lay Dying," Washington *Post,* April 17–21, 1983 (five-part series).

8. D. Breo, "Brain Surgery's Gentle Giant," *Sunday: The Chicago Tribune Magazine,* June 1, 1986, Sec. 10, p. 35.

9. MacIntyre, *After Virtue.*

10. P. J. Liacos, "The Saikewicz Decision: Keynote Address," in C. B. Wong and J. P. Swazey, eds., *Dilemmas of Dying: Policies and Procedures for Decisions Not to Treat* (Boston: G. K. Hall, 1981).

11. President's Commission, *Deciding to Forego Life-Sustaining Treatment.*

12. Pellegrino, "Toward a Reconstruction of Medical Morality," 32–56.

13. American Medical Association: *Current Opinions of the Judicial Council, 1981* (Chicago: American Medical Association, 1981), p. 25.

14. A. Camus, *Neither Victims Nor Executioners,* D. MacDonald, tr. (New York: Continuum, 1980), p. 57.

15. W. Osler, "The Old Humanities and the New Science," *Presidential Address to the Classical Association: May 16, 1919* (Boston: Houghton Mifflin, 1920), pp. 63–64.

CHAPTER 11

1. Culver and Gert, *Philosophy in Medicine.*

2. L. J. Henderson, "Physician and Patient as a Social System," *New England Journal of Medicine,* Vol. 212, No. 18 (1935), 819.

3. W. R. Houston, "The Doctor Himself as Therapeutic Agent," *Annals of Internal Medicine,* Vol. 11, No. 8 (1938), 1416–1425.
4. A. S. Ginsberg, *Decision Analysis in Clinical Patient Management with an Application to the Pleural Effusion Syndrome* (Santa Monica, Calif: Rand Corporation, 1971), p. 11.
5. H. Raiffa, *Decision Analysis: Introductory Lectures on Choices Under Uncertainty* (Reading, Mass: Addison-Wesley, 1968).
6. R. L. Keeney and H. Raiffa, *Decisions with Multiple Objections: Preferences and Value Tradeoffs* (New York: John Wiley, 1976).
7. G. W. Torrance, W. H. Thomas, and D. L. Sackett, "A Utility Maximization Model for Evaluation of Health Care Programs," *Health Services Research,* Vol. 7, No. 2 (1972), 118–133.
8. J. C. Van Es, "Medische besliskunde," *Medische Contract,* Vol. 9 (1984), 263.
9. I. Vertinsky, W. Thompson, and D. Uyeno, "Measuring Consumer Desire for Participation in Clinical Decision-Making," *Health Services Research,* Vol. 9, No. 2 (1974), 121–134.
10. T. S. Szasz and M. H. Hollender, "A Contribution to the Philosophy of Medicine: The Basic Model of the Doctor-Patient Relationship," *Archives of Internal Medicine,* Vol. 97 (1956), 585–592.
11. J. Bergsma, "Loyaal met de patient," 202–211.
12. L. R. Goldberg, "Man vs. Model of Man," *Psychiatric Bulletin,* Vol. 73 (1970), 422–432.
13. A. Tversky and D. Kahneman, "Judgment Under Uncertainty: Heuristics and Biases," *Science,* Vol. 185, No. 4157 (1974), 1124–1131.
14. P. Glover and S. Lichtenstein, "Comparison of Bayesian and Regression Approaches to the Study of Information Processing in Judgment," *Journal of Behaviour and Human Performance,* Vol. 6 (1971), 649–654.
15. W. B. Schwartz, "Decision Analysis: A Look at the Chief Complaints," *New England Journal of Medicine,* Vol. 300, No. 10 (1979), 556–559.
16. S. G. Pauker and J. P. Kassirer, "The Threshold Approach to Clinical Decision Making," *New England Journal of Medicine,* Vol. 302, No. 20 (1980), 1109–1117.
17. S. G. Pauker and J. P. Kassirer, "Clinical Application of Decision Analysis: A Detailed Illustration," *Seminars in Nuclear Medicine,* Vol. 8, No. 4 (1978), 327.
18. S. G. Pauker, "Coronary Artery Surgery: The Use of Decision Analysis," *Annals of Internal Medicine,* Vol. 85, No. 1 (1976), 8–18.
19. S. P. Pauker and S. G. Pauker, "Prenatal Diagnosis: A Directive Approach to Genetic Counseling Using Decision Analysis," *Yale Journal of Biology and Medicine,* Vol. 50, No. 3 (1977), 275–289.
20. M. C. Weinstein et al., *Clinical Decision Analysis* (Philadelphia: W. B. Saunders, 1980).
21. A. S. Brett, "Hidden Ethical Issues in Clinical Decision Analysis," *New England Journal of Medicine,* Vol. 305, No. 19 (1981), 1150–1152.
22. B. J. McNeil, R. Weichselbaum, and S. G. Pauker, "Fallacy of the Five-Year Survival in Lung Cancer," *New England Journal of Medicine,* Vol. 299, No. 25 (1978), 1397.
23. B. J. McNeil, R. Weichselbaum, and S. G. Pauker, "Speech and Survival: Tradeoffs Between Quality and Quantity of Life in Laryngeal Cancer," *New England Journal of Medicine,* Vol. 305, No. 17 (1981), 987.
24. B. McNeil, E. Keeler, and S. Adelstein, "Primer on Certain Elements of Medical Decision Making," *New England Journal of Medicine,* Vol. 293, No. 5 (1975), 211–215.

25. R. Beck, J. Kassirer, and S. Pauker, "The Convenience Approximation of Life Expectancy (the 'Deale')," *American Journal of Medicine,* Vol. 73, No. 6 (1982), 896.
26. D. Habeck, "Bedurfnis und Befreidigung des Umgangs mit Medizinischen Informationen," *Metamedicine,* Vol. 1 (1977), 237–265.
27. W. Schain, "Patients' Rights in Decision Making: The Case for Personalism Versus Paternalism in Health Care," *Cancer,* Vol. 46, No. 4 (1980), 1037.
28. W. May, "Who Cares for the Elderly?" 31–37.
29. J. Vaupel, "Structuring an Ethical Decision Dilemma," *Soundings,* Vol. 58, No. 4 (1975), 506–524.
30. A. Tversky and D. Kahneman, "The Framing of Decisions and the Psychology of Choice," *Science,* Vol. 211, No. 4481 (1981), 453–458.
31. D. Self, "A Study of the Foundation of Ethical Decision-Making of Physicians," *Theoretical Medicine,* Vol. 4, No. 1 (1983), 57–69.
32. D. Self, "Philosophical Foundations of Various Approaches to Medical Ethical Decision Making," *Journal of Medicine and Philosophy,* Vol. 4, No. 1 (1979), 10–31.
33. D. Self, "Clarification of the Philosophical Foundations for Medical Ethical Decision-Making," *Journal of Medicine and Philosophy,* Vol. 5, No. 3 (1980), 234–235.
34. D. Altman, "Statistics and Ethics in Medical Research," *British Medical Journal,* Vol. 281, No. 6249 (1980), 1182.
35. P. P. Morgan, "Clinical Trials on Trial: Must We Always Do a Randomized Trial?" *Canadian Medical Association Journal,* Vol. 125, No. 12 (1981), 1309–1311.
36. J. Henahan, "Serious Flaws Mar Many Cancer Therapy Trials," *Journal of the American Medical Association,* Vol. 250, No. 23 (1983), 3142–3143.
37. S. M. Gore, "Assessing Clinical Trials: First Steps," *British Medical Journal,* Vol. 282, No. 6276 (1981), 1605–1607.
38. S. Levitt, "The Role of Radiation Therapy in the Treatment of Breast Cancer: The Use and Abuse of Clinical Trials, Statistics and Unproven Hypotheses," *International Journal of Radiation Oncology, Biology and Physics,* Vol. 6, No. 7 (1980), 791–798.
39. D. P. Byar, "Sound Advice for Conducting Clinical Trials," *New England Journal of Medicine,* Vol. 297, No. 10 (1977), 553–554.
40. S. Schor and I. Karten, "Statistical Evaluation of Medical Journal Manuscripts," *Journal of the American Medical Association,* Vol. 195, No. 13 (1966), 1123–1128.
41. D. L. Sackett, "Bias in Analytic Research," *Journal of Chronic Diseases,* Vol. 32, Nos. 1/2 (1979), 51–63.
42. J. C. Holland, "Patients Who Seek Unproven Cancer Remedies: A Psychological Perspective," *Clinical Bulletin,* Vol. 11 (1981), 102–105.
43. P. Arkko et al., "A Survey of Unproven Cancer Remedies and Their Uses in an Outpatient Clinic for Cancer Therapy in Finland," *Social Science and Medicine,* Vol. 14a, No. 6 (1980), 511–514.
44. Letters to the editor, "A New Design for Randomized Trials," *New England Journal of Medicine,* Vol. 301, No. 14 (1979), 786–788.
45. G. M. Lawrie and M. E. DeBakey, "The Coronary Artery Surgery Study," *Journal of the American Medical Association,* Vol. 252, No. 18 (1984), 2609–2611.
46. D. L. Sackett and R. W. Torrance, "The Utility of Different Health States as Perceived by the General Public," *Journal of Chronic Disease,* Vol. 31 (1978), 697–704.
47. E. H. Morreim, "Three Concepts of Patient Competence," *Theoretical Medicine,* Vol. 4, No. 3 (1983), 231–251.
48. W. St. C. Symmers, "Not Allowed to Die," *British Medical Journal,* Vol. 1, No. 5589 (1968), 442.

49. J. E. Wendte, *Patienten in het ziekenhuis* (Amsterdam: Rodopi, 1984).
50. B. J. Volicer and M. W. Bohannon, "A Hospital Stress Relating Scale," *Nursing Research,* Vol. 24, No. 5 (1975), 352–359.
51. S. J. Youngner and D. L. Jackson, "Family Wishes and Patient Autonomy," *Hastings Center Report,* Vol. 7, No. 5 (1980), 21–22.
52. J. Katz and A. Capron, *"Catastrophic Disease: Who Decides What?* (New York: Russell Sage Foundation, 1975).
53. Siegler, "Critical Illness," 12–15.
54. Cassell, "The Function of Medicine," 16–19.
55. E. Baumgarten, "The Concept of 'Competence' in Medical Ethics," *Journal of Medical Ethics,* Vol. 6, No. 4 (1980), 180–184.
56. D. Callahan, "On Defining a 'Natural Death,'" *Hastings Center Report,* Vol. 7, No. 3 (1977), 32–37.
57. J. Blits, "Natural Death and Moral Individuality," *Journal of Medical Ethics,* Vol. 5, No. 3 (1980), 236–245.
58. D. Thomasma, "Ethical Judgments of Quality of Life in the Care of the Aged," *Journal of the American Geriatrics Society,* Vol. 37, No. 7 (1984), 525–527.
59. C. B. Cohen, " 'Quality of Life,' and the Analogy with the Nazis," *Journal of Medicine and Philosophy,* Vol. 8, No. 2 (1983), 114.
60. R. W. Momeyer, "Medical Decisions Concerning Noncompetent Patients," *Theoretical Medicine,* Vol. 4, No. 3 (1983), 275–290.
61. S. Gadow, "Medicine, Ethics, and the Elderly," *The Gerontologist,* Vol. 20, No. 6 (1980), 683.

CHAPTER 12

1. C. Culver and B. Gert, *Philosophy in Medicine: Conceptual and Ethical Issues.* (New York: Oxford University Press, 1982).
2. D. Wikler, "Paternalism and the Mildly Retarded," *Philosophy and Public Affairs,* Vol. 8, No. 4 (1979), 377–392.
3. T. L. Beauchamp and L. B. McCullough, *Medical Ethics: The Moral Responsibilities of Physicians* (Englewood Cliffs, NJ: Prentice-Hall, 1984), pp. 118–128.
4. President's Commission, *Making Health Care Decisions.*
5. Beauchamp and McCullough, *Medical Ethics,* pp. 118–128.
6. See articles by E. H. Morreim, T. Beauchamp, E. Pincoffs, and J. Knight in E. Shelp, H. T. Englehardt, Jr., and S. Spicker, eds., *Philosophy and Medicine* (Dordrecht: D. Reidel, in press).
7. R. B. White and H. T. Engelhardt, Jr., "A Demand to Die," *Hastings Center Report,* Vol. 5, No. 3 (1975), 9–10.
8. Jackson and Youngner, "Patient Autonomy," 404–408.
9. M. Siegler, "Critical Illness: The Limits of Autonomy," *Hastings Center Report,* Vol. 7, No. 5 (1977), 12–15.
10. Childress, *Who Should Decide?* pp. 63–65; 103–107.
11. Siegler, "Critical Illness," 12–15.
12. Youngner and Jackson, "Family Wishes and Patient Autonomy," 21–22.
13. Pellegrino, "Being Ill and Being Healed," 70–79.
14. M. Siegler, "Commentary: Does Doing Everything Include CPR?" *Hastings Center Report,* Vol. 12, No. 5 (1982), 27–29.
15. Beauchamp and McCullough, *Medical Ethics,* pp. 118–128.

16. L. H. Roth, A. Meisel, and C. Lidz, "Tests of Competency to Consent to Treatment," *American Journal of Psychiatry,* Vol. 134, No. 3 (1977), 279–285.
17. Beauchamp and McCullough, *Medical Ethics,* pp. 118–128.
18. Ibid.
19. Ibid., pp. 132.
20. Ackerman, "Fooling Ourselves with Child Autonomy," 345–348.
21. J. S. Mill, *On Liberty,* G. Himmelfarb, ed. (New York: Penguin, 1974), pp. 68–69.
22. *Schloendorff v. The Society of New York Hospitals,* 211 N.Y. 127, 129; 105 N.E. 92, 93 (1914).
23. *Natanson v. Kline,* 186 Kan. 393; 350 P. 2d 1093 (1960).
24. *Bartling v. Superior Court; Bartling v. Glendale Adventist Medical Center.*
25. President's Commission, *Making Health Care Decisions.*
26. J. F. Drane, "Competency to Give an Informed Consent," *Journal of the American Medical Association,* Vol. 252, No. 7 (1984), 925–927. This paper calls for a sliding scale of criteria for competency.
27. J. Knight, "Judging Competence: When the Psychiatrist Need or Need Not Be Involved," in H. T. Engelhardt, Jr., M. A. Gardell, and E. E. Shelp, eds., *When Are Competent Patients Incompetent?* (Dordrecht: D. Reidel, in press).
28. See B. Stanley et al., "The Elderly Patient and Informed Consent," *Journal of the American Medical Association,* Vol. 252, No. 10 (1984), 1302–1306. Empirical data are provided to show that elderly patients' choices are as reasonable as those of younger patients, even though their comprehension of consent information is significantly less. Here is an example in which the physician's obligation to enhance competence must center on enhancing comprehension.

CHAPTER 13

1. C. Hackler, R. Moseley, and D. Vawter, eds., *Advance Directives* (Philadelphia: Praeger, in press).
2. Cf. *Theoretical Medicine* Vol. 7, No. 2 (1986). The focus of this issue is "The Physician's Influence on Patient Decision Making."
3. Veatch, *Death, Dying and the Biological Revolution.*
4. See the discussion of this problem in T. Swick, "Interpreting the Quinlan Decision 10 Years After," *American College of Physicians Observer,* Vol. 6 (June 1986), 18, 22.
5. Stollerman, "Promoting Patient Autonomy," 9–15.
6. *Schloendorff v. The Society of New York Hospitals.*
7. President's Commission, *Deciding to Forego Life-Sustaining Treatment,* p. 3.
8. Siegler, "Searching for Moral Certainty," 57–69.
9. Jonsen, Siegler, and Winslade, *Clinical Ethics,* pp. 55–56.
10. G. Weiss, "Paternalism Modernised," *Journal of Medical Ethics,* Vol. 11, No. 4 (1985), 184–187. Also see Childress and Siegler, "Metaphors and Models of Doctor-Patient Relationships," 17–30.
11. "Living Will Invites Patient-Physician Dialogue," *Frontlines,* Vol. 2, No. 2 (1985), 1.
12. American Medical Association Council on Ethical and Judicial Affairs, "Revised Statement on Life-Prolonging Treatment," *American Medical Association News,* Vol. 29, No. 12 (1986).
13. *In the Matter of Claire C. Conroy.*
14. "Doctor on Trial in 'Right to Die' Case," New York *Times* (September 19, 1985), Sec. 1, p. 24.

15. One of the first physicians to decry preserving life at all costs was Ralph Crawshaw. He relates the tale of a colleague's brother, who suffered greatly from multiple myeloma, and an aggressive nephrologist, who stubbornly refused even to discuss withholding treatment while running up a bill of forty-seven thousand dollars. Crawshaw ends his article with harsh criticism of medical zealotry. R. Crawshaw, "Technical Zeal and Therapeutic Purpose: How to Decide?" *Journal of the American Medical Association,* Vol. 250, No. 14 (1983), 1857–1859.
16. D. Thomasma, "Hospital Ethics Committees: Laying the Groundwork," *Bioethics Reporter,* Vol. 3 (1985), 381.
17. M. Siegler, "Ethics Committees: Decisions by Bureaucracy," *Hastings Center Report,* Vol. 16, No. 3 (1986), 22–24.
18. *Elizabeth Bouvia v. Superior Court (Glenchur).*
19. Engelhardt, *The Foundations of Bioethics.*
20. R. A. Burt, "Immunizing Physicians by Law," in C. B. Wang and J. P. Swazey, eds., *Dilemmas in Dying* (Boston: G. K. Hall, 1981), p. 147.
21. Ibid., p. 148.
22. "In the Matter of the Treatment and Care of Infant Doe," declaratory judgment. *Connecticut Medicine,* Vol. 47, No. 7 (1983), 409–410.
23. *In the matter of William E. Weber, guardian ad litem for Baby Jane Doe v. Stony Brook Hospital, et al.,* 456 N.E. 2d 1186; 467 N.E. 2d 685.
24. Department of Health and Human Services, "Child Abuse and Neglect Prevention and Treatment Program," *Federal Register,* Vol. 49 (1984), 1622–1654, and *Federal Register,* Vol. 50 (1985), 14873–14892. Also see J. Moskop and R. Saldanha, "The Brief but Stormy History of Federal Intervention," *Hastings Center Report,* Vol. 16, No. 2 (1986), 10–11.

CHAPTER 14

1. Fees for service—in goods, preferments, or money—are as old as medicine. Fees, their level, problems in collection, and the like are found in many of the books of the Hippocratic corpus.
2. Plato *Republic,* I, 342d.
3. Ibid., I, 346b.
4. Ibid., I, 346d.
5. G. B. Shaw, *The Doctor's Dilemma* (Baltimore: Penguin, 1965). Note especially the acerbic but, sadly, too often accurate, "Preface on Doctors."
6. Cushing, *Consecratio Medici,* pp. 3–13. Also see E. D. Pellegrino, "What Is a Profession?" *Journal of Allied Health,* Vol. 12, No. 3 (1983), 168–176.
7. The Hippocratic oath is still the most common public declaration of voluntary assumption of ethical obligations inherent in medicine. Other oaths, such as the so-called oath of Maimonides, the oath of Geneva, and the World Health Organization, all carry the same message of commitment to the good of others. This is true of the oath of the Soviet physicians as well, with one significant difference we shall comment upon later.
8. Studies of experiences with physician gatekeeping are beginning to appear. Examples of such studies are these: J. M. Eisenberg, "The Internist as Gatekeeper," *Annals of Internal Medicine,* Vol. 102, No. 4 (1985), 537–543; A. R. Somers, "And Who Shall Be the Gatekeeper? The Role of the Primary Physician in the Health Care Delivery System," *Inquiry,* Vol. 20, No. 4 (1983), 301–313; J. K. Inglehart, "Medicaid Turns

to Prepaid Managed Care," *New England Journal of Medicine,* Vol. 308, No. 16 (1983), 976–980; and S. H. Moore, "Cost Containment Through Risk Sharing by Primary Care Physicians," *New England Journal of Medicine,* Vol. 300, No. 24 (1979), 1359–1362.

9. U. Reinhardt, "Health and Hot Potatoes," editorial, Washington *Post,* March 16, 1985, sec. A, p. 20.

10. AARP hot line for insurance and information: 1-800-523-5800.

11. R. Kotulak, "Program to Cut Medicaid Cost May Hurt Poor," Chicago *Tribune,* Sunday, March 9, 1986, sec. 2, pp. 1–2.

12. Some of the tendencies, dangers, and conflicts potentially harmful to patients and ethically suspect are discussed in the following: R. A. Rosenblatt and I. S. Moscovice, "The Physician as Gatekeeper," *Medical Care,* Vol. 22, No. 2 (1984), 150–159; A. S. Relman, "The Allocation of Medical Resources by Physicians," *Journal of Medical Education,* Vol. 55 No. 2 (1980), 99–104; S. H. Moore, D. Martin, and W. C. Richardson, "Does the Primary Gatekeeper Control the Costs of Health Care?" *New England Journal of Medicine,* Vol. 309 No. 22 (1983), 1400–1404; and B. F. Overholt, "The Socioeconomic and Political Future of Gastroenterology. Part II: Primary Care Network—The Gatekeeper," *American Journal of Gastroenterology,* Vol. 78, No. 7 (1983), 456–460.

13. W. B. Schwartz and H. J. Aaron, "Rationing Hospital Care: Lessons from Britain," *New England Journal of Medicine,* Vol. 310, No. 4 (1984), 52–56.

14. P. W. Butler, R. C. Bone, and T. Field, "Technology Under Medicare Diagnosis-Related Groups Prospective Payment: Implications for Medical Intensive Care," *Chest,* Vol. 87, No. 2 (1985), 229–234.

15. Department of Health and Human Services, *Summary Report of the Graduate Medical Education National Advisory Committee to the Secretary* (Washington, DC: U.S. Government Printing Office, 1980).

16. P. Starr, *The Social Transformation of American Medicine* (New York: Basic Books, 1982).

17. Pellegrino, "Toward a Reconstruction of Medical Morality," 32–56.

18. G. Calabresi and P. Bobbitt, *Tragic Choices* (New York: W. W. Norton, 1978).

19. R. Catlin, R. C. Bradbury, and R. J. O. Catlin, "Primary Care Gatekeepers in HMO's," *The Journal of Family Practice,* Vol. 17, No. 4 (1983), 673–678.

20. P. Dans, J. P. Weiner, and S. Otter, "Peer Review Organizations: Promises and Potential Pitfalls," *New England Journal of Medicine,* Vol. 313, No. 18 (1985), 1131–1137.

21. J. C. Moskop, "The Moral Limits to Federal Funding for Kidney Disease," *Hastings Center Report* Vol. 17, No. 2 (1987), 11–15.

22. Figures for national expenditures for goods, commodities, and services are difficult to evaluate. For our purposes the important point is the relative order of magnitude of specific health and medical care expenditures as compared with other expenditures. See each year's July issue of the U.S. Department of Commerce *Survey of Current Business* and also *U.S. Statistical Abstracts* for these figures.

23. D. Thomasma, "Advance Directives and Elder Care," in *The Arkansas Conference on the Society for Health and Human Values: Proceedings,* (unpublished).

24. American College of Surgeons. See also I. M. Rutkow, "Unnecessary Surgery: What Is It?" *Surgical Clinics of North America,* Vol. 62, No. 4 (1982), 613–625; I. M. Rutkow, "Rates of Surgery in the United States: The Decade of the 1970s," *Surgical Clinics of North America,* Vol. 62, No. 4 (1982), 559–578; and G. Zuidema, *The Study on Surgical Services for the United States* (Baltimore: Lewis, 1975).

25. Debates about the nature of justice and the principles of distributive justice that should obtain are particularly active today. See J. Rawls, *A Theory of Justice* (Cambridge: Harvard University Press, 1971); and R. Nozick, *Anarchy, State and Utopia* (New York: Basic Books, 1974).

26. Most of the litigation is still in the possible state being underlined by lawyers in informal opinions that are probably well grounded. For example, see A. R. Chenen, "Prospective Payment Can Put You in Court," *Medical Economics,* July 9, 1984, 134ff.; W. H. Ginsburg, "DRG's: Must Physicians and Hospitals Be Adversaries?" *Physician's Management,* Vol. 25, No. 5 (1985), 292ff.; and P. Gerber, "How DRG's Increase Your Malpractice Risk," *Physician's Management,* Vol. 24, No. 2 (1985), 335ff. Also see W. J. Curran, "Economic and Legal Considerations in Emergency Care for Analysis of the Case of *Thompson v. Sun City Community Hospital,*" *New England Journal of Medicine,* Vol. 312, No. 6 (1985), 374–375. In this case a young boy needing emergency surgery was transferred for financial reasons in a "stable" state. Suit was brought by the patient's mother against the hospital, the emergency room, and the physician for permanent impairment resulting from delay in surgery. The court found against the hospital but not the physician. More cases of this type surely can be anticipated, and physician liability will surely be questioned in each.

27. E. D. Pellegrino, "Rationing Health Care: The Ethics of Medical Gatekeeping," *Journal of Contemporary Health Law Policy,* Vol. 2 (1986), 23–45.

28. R. L. Schiff et al., "Special Article: Transfers to a Public Hospital: A Prospective Study of 467 Patients," *New England Journal of Medicine,* Vol. 314, No. 9 (1986), 552–557.

29. Matt. 6:24.

CHAPTER 15

1. *In the matter of Karen Quinlan,* 70 N.J. 10, 44; 355 A. 2d 647; cert. den., 429 U.S. 922; 50 L. Ed. 2d 289 (N.J. 1976).

2. *Superintendent of Belchertown State School v. Saikewicz* 373 Mass. 738; 370 NE 2d 417, 424 (1977).

3. H. W. Classen, "The Doctrine of Substituted Judgment in Its Medicolegal Context," *Medical Trial Technique Quarterly,* Vol. 31 (1985), 451–467.

4. J. R. Connery, "Court's Guidelines on Incompetent Patients Compromise Their Rights," *Hospital Progress,* Vol. 61, No. 9 (1980), 46–49.

5. A. S. Relman, "The Saikewicz Decision: Judges as Physicians," *New England Journal of Medicine,* Vol. 298, No. 9 (1978), 508.

6. L. S. Routhenburg, "The Empty Search for an Imprimatur, or Delphic Oracles Are in Short Supply," *Law, Medicine and Health Care,* Vol. 10 (1982), 115, note 3.

7. Department of Health and Human Services, "Child Abuse and Neglect Prevention and Treatment Program," *Federal Register,* Vol. 49 (1984), 1622–1654 and *Federal Register,* Vol. 50 (1985), 14873–14892.

8. *Barber and Nejdl v. Superior Court of State of California* 195 Cal. Rptr. 484; 147 Cal. App. 3d 1054 (1983).

9. G. R. Ginex, "A Prosecutor's View on Criminal Liability for Withholding or Withdrawing Medical Care," in A. E. Doudera and J. D. Peters, eds. *Legal and Ethical Aspects of Treating Critically and Terminally Ill Patients* (Ann Arbor, Mich: Aupha Press), pp. 205–210.

10. G. Kelly, "The Duty of Using Artificial Means of Preserving Life," *Theological Studies,* Vol. 11, No. 2 (1950), 203–220.

11. J. J. McCartney, "The Development of the Doctrine of Ordinary and Extraordinary Means of Preserving Life in Catholic Moral Theology Before the Karen Quinlan Case," *Linacre Quarterly,* Vol. 47, No. 3 (1980), 215–224.
12. D. C. Thomasma, K. C. Micetich, and P. H. Steinecker, "Continuance of Care in the Terminally Ill Patient," *Clinics in Critical Care,* Vol. 2, No. 1 (1986), 61–71.
13. David T. Watts and C. K. Cassell, "Extraordinary Nutritional Support," *Journal of the American Geriatrics Society,* Vol. 32, No. 3 (1984), 237–242.
14. Often the intravenous lines are left in at a "keep-open rate," more to assuage the physician's conscience than to benefit the patient. See K. Micetich, P. Steinecker, and D. Thomasma, "Are Intravenous Fluids Morally Required for a Dying Patient?" *Archives of Internal Medicine,* Vol. 143, No. 5 (1983), 975–978.
15. "Opinion of the AMA Council on Ethical and Judicial Affairs; Withholding or Withdrawing Life-Prolonging Medical Treatment," *American Medical Association News,* Vol. 29, No. 12 (1986), 1.
16. "In the Matter of the Treatment and Care of Infant Doe," 409–410.
17. *In the matter of William A. Weber, guardian ad litem for Baby Jane Doe v. Stony Brook Hospital et al.*
18. D. Thomasma, "An Interdisciplinary Code for Team Care," *Proceedings of the Ninth Annual Interdisciplinary Health Care Conference.* Presentation delivered September 19, 1986, Ohio State University, Columbus, Ohio.
19. *Bartling v. Superior Court; Bartling v. Glendale Adventist Medical Center.*
20. M. Kapp and B. Lo, "Legal Perceptions and Medical Decisionmaking," A report for the Congressional Office of Technology Assessment, Washington, DC, March, 1986, p. 27:

    The presentation of the case in the media implied that court action was the only way to resolve the disagreement. It did not present a less dramatic alternative: that agreement might be possible through improved communication between caregivers and the patient or by psychological treatments. On the one hand, Mr. Bartling might agree to treatment for his depression. On the other hand, if physicians were convinced that his refusal of treatment was truly informed and consistent, then they might be willing to accept his wishes.

21. *In the matter of Claire C. Conroy.*
22. G. Stollerman, "Lovable Decisions: Re-Humanizing Dying," *Journal of the American Geriatrics Society,* Vol. 34, No. 2 (1986), 172–174.
23. M. Nevins, "Analysis of the Supreme Court of New Jersey's Decision in the Claire Conroy Case," *Journal of the American Geriatrics Society,* Vol. 34, No. 2 (1986), 140–143.
24. *In the matter of Nancy Ellen Jobes,* Superior Court of N.J. Chancery Division, Morris County, docket no. C-4971-85E, (April 23, 1986).
25. *Patricia E. Brophy, guardian of Paul E. Brophy v. New England Sinai Hospital,* Commonwealth of Massachusetts, the Trial Court, the Probate and Family Court Department, Norfolk Division, docket no. 85E0009-GL, (October 21, 1985).
26. *In the matter of Nancy Ellen Jobes.*
27. Ibid. p. 9.
28. *In the matter of Conservatorship Torres,* 357 N.W. 2d 332 (Minn. 1984).
29. *Elizabeth Bouvia v. County of Riverside,* No. 159780, Superior Court, Riverside, California, (December 16, 1983).
30. *Elizabeth Bouvia v. Superior Court (Glenchur).*
31. Kapp and Lo, "Legal Perceptions and Medical Decisionmaking," p. 26.
32. *Elizabeth Bouvia v. Superior Court (Glenchur),* p. 22.

33. Engelhardt, *The Foundation of Bioethics.*
34. E. D. Pellegrino, "Medical Ethics," *Journal of the American Medical Association,* Vol. 256, No. 15 (1986), 2122–2124.
35. A theological basis of medical practice is also required, since philosophy itself has its limits.
36. *Corbett v. D'Allesandro,* 13th Circuit, Lee County, Florida, case no. 84-5627 CA-JRT, February 28, 1985.
37. *Corbett v. D'Allesandro,* 487 So. 2d 368 (Fla. App. 1986).
38. MacIntyre, *After Virtue.*
39. Engelhardt, *The Foundations of Bioethics.*

CHAPTER 16

1. One need only compare the seven restrained declaratory statements of the latest revision of the AMA code (*Principles of Medical Ethics,* adopted 1980) with its predecessors, the AMA code of 1847: American Medical Association, *Code of Ethics; Adopted May 1847* (Philadelphia: Collins, 1848); American Medical Association, *Code of Ethics; Adopted May 1847* (Concord: McFarland, 1850); and the revised code of 1882: American Medical Association, *Code of Ethics Adopted by the American Medical Association (Revised to Date)* (New York: William Wood, 1882). See also Percival's *Ethics* of 1794: T. Percival, *Medical Jurisprudence; or, A Code of Ethics and Institutes, Adapted to the Professions of Physic and Surgery* (Manchester: S. Russell, 1794), as well as Percival's revised ethics of 1803: T. Percival, *Ethics, or, a Code of Institutes and Precepts: Adapted to the Professional Conduct of Physicians and Surgeons* (Manchester: A. Russell, 1803), and the reprint of Percival's medical ethics: C. D. Leake, ed., *Percival's Medical Ethics* (Baltimore: Williams & Wilkins, 1927). See also The Ad Hoc Committee on Medical Ethics, American College of Physicians, "American College of Physicians Ethics Manual," Vol. 101, Nos. 1 and 2 (1984), 129–137; 263–274.
2. Pellegrino, "Toward a Reconstruction of Medical Morality," 32–56.
3. That this is not a new phenomenon is clear if one looks at the historical record of physicians' aberrant behavior: G. T. Witkowski, "Le mal quon dit des medecins," cited in C. L. Dana, "The evil spoken of physicians," *Proceedings of the Charaka Club,* Vol. 1 (1920), 77–90.
4. Veatch, *A Theory of Medical Ethics.*
5. Berlant, *Profession and Monopoly.*
6. Seneca *De Beneficis,* VI, 16.
7. Lain-Entralgo, *Doctor and Patient.*
8. H. Jonas, *The Imperative of Responsibility* (Chicago: Unviersity of Chicago Press, 1984).
9. Dr. Abrams' affirmation and ours share a similar goal and content:

A Physician's Affirmation

In order to be worthy of self-respect, I pledge to respect others who place their trust in me as a professional in the healing arts. Therefore:

I will practice my art and my science to benefit my patients.

I will *disclose* to my patients that which I know of their disease, and any hazards of the remedies I might suggest, that I may guide them to choose the course that suits them best.

I will offer care and comfort when they are ill, and when death becomes inevitable, I will ease their way as best I can in keeping with their expressed plan.

I will recognize their right to self-determination, and if conflict should arise with my own ethical constraints, make them aware without judging wherein we differ, that they should consider seeking help elsewhere for their complaints.

I will intercede in their behalf within the scope of my authority if I perceive they are being treated without regard for their humanity.

I will hold in confidence that which is seen or heard in my role as physician.

I will ever be a student to sharpen my skills and further my knowledge that I may be a better clinician.

If I act in this way I may aspire to join the men and women who, through the ages, have approached the loftiest ideals of the healing mission, for I will have earned the faith and trust which is the strongest tie in the bond between patient and physician.

(Copies can be obtained from Fred R. Abrams, M.D., Center for Applied Biomedical Ethics at Rose Medical Center, 4567 East Ninth Avenue, Denver, CO 80220.)

10. R. Napodano, *Values in Medical Practice: A Statement of Philosophy for Physicians and a Model for Teaching a Healing Science* (New York: Human Sciences Press, 1986), pp. 53–57.
11. R. Bulger, *In Search of the Modern Hippocrates* (Iowa City: University of Iowa Press, 1987).

Index